Manual of ENDOSCOPY

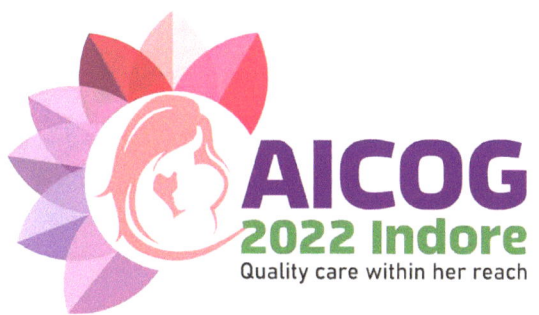

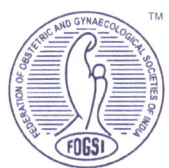 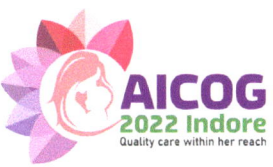 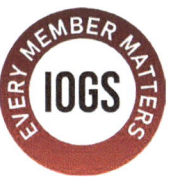 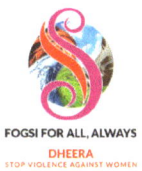

64th All India Congress of Obstetrics and Gynaecology
04–08 April 2022

Manual of
ENDOSCOPY
Cutting Edge

Editors

Asha Baxi
MS FICOG FRCOG
Chief Consultant
Dr Asha Baxi's Fertility Centre
Motherhood Hospital
Indore, Madhya Pradesh, India

Dhaval Baxi
MBBS DGO DNB MCh
(Reproductive Medicine & Surgery)
Consultant Gynecologist
Endoscopic Surgeon and
Fertility Specialist
Disha Fertility and Surgical Centre
Motherhood Hospital
Indore, Madhya Pradesh, India

Co-Editors

Archana Dubey
MBBS MS (OBG)
Consultant-Gynecologist
Infertility and Laparoscopy
Motherhood Hospital
Indore, Madhya Pradesh, India

Astha Jain Mathur
MBBS DGO
Chief Consultant
Consultant-Obstetrician and
Gynecologist
Motherhood Hospital
Indore, Madhya Pradesh, India

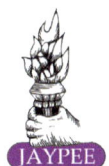

JAYPEE BROTHERS MEDICAL PUBLISHERS
The Health Sciences Publisher
New Delhi | London

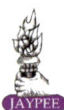 **Jaypee Brothers Medical Publishers (P) Ltd.**

Headquarters
Jaypee Brothers Medical Publishers (P) Ltd
EMCA House, 23/23-B
Ansari Road, Daryaganj
New Delhi 110 002, India
Landline: +91-11-23272143, +91-11-23272703
+91-11-23282021, +91-11-23245672
Email: jaypee@jaypeebrothers.com

Corporate Office
Jaypee Brothers Medical Publishers (P) Ltd
4838/24, Ansari Road, Daryaganj
New Delhi 110 002, India
Phone: +91-11-43574357
Fax: +91-11-43574314
Email: jaypee@jaypeebrothers.com

Overseas Office
JP Medical Ltd.
83, Victoria Street, London
SW1H 0HW (UK)
Phone: +44 20 3170 8910
Fax: +44 (0)20 3008 6180
Email: info@jpmedpub.com

Website: www.jaypeebrothers.com
Website: www.jaypeedigital.com

© 2022, Jaypee Brothers Medical Publishers

The views and opinions expressed in this book are solely those of the original contributor(s)/author(s) and do not necessarily represent those of editor(s) of the book.

All rights reserved. No part of this publication may be reproduced, stored or transmitted in any form or by any means, electronic, mechanical, photocopying, recording or otherwise, without the prior permission in writing of the publishers.

All brand names and product names used in this book are trade names, service marks, trademarks or registered trademarks of their respective owners. The publisher is not associated with any product or vendor mentioned in this book.

Medical knowledge and practice change constantly. This book is designed to provide accurate, authoritative information about the subject matter in question. However, readers are advised to check the most current information available on procedures included and check information from the manufacturer of each product to be administered, to verify the recommended dose, formula, method and duration of administration, adverse effects and contraindications. It is the responsibility of the practitioner to take all appropriate safety precautions. Neither the publisher nor the author(s)/editor(s) assume any liability for any injury and/or damage to persons or property arising from or related to use of material in this book.

This book is sold on the understanding that the publisher is not engaged in providing professional medical services. If such advice or services are required, the services of a competent medical professional should be sought.

Every effort has been made where necessary to contact holders of copyright to obtain permission to reproduce copyright material. If any have been inadvertently overlooked, the publisher will be pleased to make the necessary arrangements at the first opportunity. The **CD/DVD-ROM** (if any) provided in the sealed envelope with this book is complimentary and free of cost. **Not meant for sale.**

Inquiries for bulk sales may be solicited at: jaypee@jaypeebrothers.com

Manual of Endoscopy

First Edition: **2022**

ISBN: 978-93-5465-683-5

Printed at Repro India Limited

Dedicated to
Gynecologists and women worldwide.

Contributors

Aditi Abhade MBBS MS
Junior Consultant
Department of Obstetrics and
Gynecology
JK Women Hospital
Dombivli, Maharashtra, India

Asha Baxi
MS FICOG FRCOG
Chief Consultant
Dr Asha Baxi's Fertility Centre
Motherhood Hospital
Indore, Madhya Pradesh, India

Anshu Baser MS DNB
Consultant
Akash Hospital and Diagnostic Centre
Indore, Madhya Pradesh, India

Archana Baser
MS DNB FRCOG FICOG
Consultant
Obstetrician and Gynecologist
Director, Akash Hospital
Indore, Madhya Pradesh, India

Archana Dubey
MBBS MS (OBG)
Consultant-Gynecologist
Infertility and Laparoscopy
Motherhood Hospital
Indore, Madhya Pradesh, India

Astha Jain Mathur MBBS DGO
Chief Consultant
Consultant-Obstetrician and
Gynaecologist
Motherhood Hospital
Indore, Madhya Pradesh, India

B Ramesh
MBBS MD DGO FCPS Diploma in Gyne
Endoscopy (Atlanta, USA) PhD in
Urogynecology
Gyne Laparosurgeon
IVF Specialist and Urogynecologist
Medical Director and Chief
Laparoscopic Surgeon
Altius Hospitals Pvt Ltd
Bengaluru, Karnataka, India

Damodar Rao
MBBS MD FICOG FIMG FRM FMAS
Associate Director, Rao Hospital
Consultant, Infertility and Laparoscopy
Coimbatore, Tamil Nadu, India

Dhaval Baxi
MBBS DGO DNB MCh (Reproductive Medicine
& Surgery)
Consultant Gynecologist
Endoscopic Surgeon and
Fertility Specialist
Disha Fertility and Surgical Centre
Motherhood Hospital
Indore, Madhya Pradesh, India

Jasmine S Abraham MBBS MS
Obstetrician Gynec Endoscopy and
Infertility
Altius Hospital
Bengaluru, Karnataka, India

Manjula Anagani MD FICOG
Padmashree Awardee
Clinical Director and Head
Infertility Specialist and Laparoscopic
Surgeon
Maxcure Hospitals
Hyderabad, Telangana, India

Contributors

Pandit Palaskar
MBBS MD DNBE DFP MNAMS Diploma in Endoscopic Surgery (Australia)
Gynecological Endoscopic Surgeon
IVF-ICSI Infertility Specialist
Endoworld Hospital
Aurangabad, Maharashtra, India

R Sindura Ganga MS
Gynecologist and Obstetrics
Laparoscopic Surgeon
Suyosha Clinic
Hyderabad, Telangana, India

S Krishnakumar MD DGO
Chief Consultant
JK Women Hospital, Mumbai
Fortis Hospital, Kalyan, Mumbai
Immediate Past President
Indian Association of Gynaecological Endoscopists

Subash Mallya MBBS DGO DNB MNAMS
Diploma in Endoscopy (Germany)
Consultant Gyne Endoscopy Surgeon
Baby Memorial Hospital and PVS
Hospital, Calicut, Kerala, India

Swathi HV MS
Obstetrician and Gynecologist
COG Fellow of Gyn Laparoscopy
Care Hospital
Hyderabad, Telangana, India

Yashodhan Deka MS DNB FMAS FIAGE
Consultant
Endoscopic Surgeon
Sarathi Hospital
Nalbari, Assam, India

Vivek Salunke MD
Gyne Endoscopy Surgeon
Nalini Speciality Hospital
Mumbai, Maharashtra, India

Message

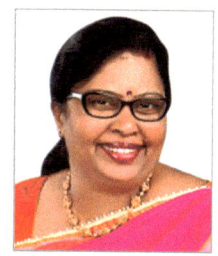 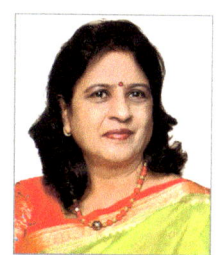

S Shantha Kumari **Madhuri Patel**
President, FOGSI   Secretary General, FOGSI

Dear delegates
Dil se Namaste
Warm greetings!

On behalf of the organizing committee, I would like to welcome you all to our prestigious national conference—AICOG 2022.

This is being held after a gap of 2 long years. Long because of the uncertainties, hitherto unknown unprecedented road-blocks created by the scourge of the humanity COVID-19.

We are aware of the hard work and dedication of the Indore team. The way they have kept up their spirits is commendable.

As we move ahead in our path of scientific advances, we must ensure that it reaches out to the masses. Hence the theme of the conference "Quality Care within her Reach."

These workshops have been planned meticulously for you all to feast upon and enrich yourself with additional knowledge.

It has always been the endeavor of FOGSI to strive to impart knowledge with camaraderie and bonhomie, and both of us, wish you the very best.

Message from Organizing Committee

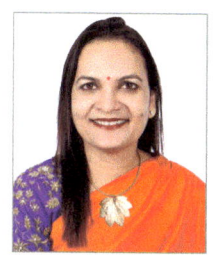 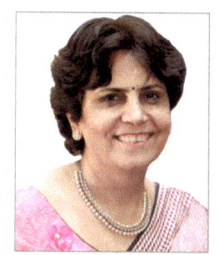 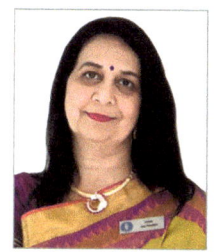

Asha Baxi
Organizing President

Kawita Bapat
Organizing Secretary

Archana Baser
Organizing Secretary

Dear All
Pranam, Namaste, and Swagatam
Welcome and Warm Greetings!

On behalf of the organizing committee, it gives us immense happiness to heartily welcome each one of you, to this revered prestigious National Conference of AICOG 2022.

Madhya Pradesh is the heart of India, and Indore being its 'Dil' become the warmest and cleanest place to welcome you all.

We as a team, will try our best, that you always have memories to cherish forever of this conference.

The Ob/Gyn fraternity of the whole of Madhya Pradesh, stands with solidarity to ensure you have an academic feast, to titillate/stimulate your brain.

The course of planning of AICOG 2022, was a tough one. We were always swinging with the pendulum of the time, very unsure of the feasibility of conference. The waxing and waning of COVID, made our preparations reach either acme or nadir.

Despite the hurdles, we are bound to enthrall you with a scientific bonanza rolled out. Scientific advances never stop with any pandemic or calamity.

We wish that you keep abreast of all the latest advances, be it in the management of the dreaded COVID in pregnancy, ART, vaginal surgeries, oncology, endoscopy, cosmetic and uro-gynecology, or ultrasound and fetal medicine.

After great deliberation, discussion and brainstorming, we finalized 8 Pre-congress Workshops on 9th January 2022; with live demonstrations, video presentations, interactive teachings and the thrills of drills, to ensure that you go back enriched and enthralled.

Youngsters have a comprehensive package of Obstetrics in the "Beginners Delights" from 'foundation' to the 'crescendo' learning the finer nuances of the practice of Ob/Gyn.

The advances in medicine and the easy availability of the Internet knowledge, has lead to dwindling patient-doctor faith and increasing unfound conflicts. As a gynecologist, it is our moral responsibility to ensure not only the physical, but 'mental and emotional' health of the woman.

Thus we have a separate workshop addressing these medicolegal issues such as the latest amendment in the MTP Act, POCSO Act, VAW (Dheera) Act, examination of a survivor, apart from interactive sessions on actual cases. You can spruce up your knowledge with experts of the field.

The theme of the conference is "Quality Care within her Reach", and it is our utmost endeavor to enrich you with the ability to impart quality care with humanity and humility.

The workshops are chosen with extreme conscious efforts to meet the highest academic standards in a limited time, and I am confident that you shall enjoy the limited overs match hugely.

We are looking forward to welcoming you to the wonderful city of Malwa, Indore. The city known for its culture, hospitality, unique Cusine and of course the cleanliness.

So do join us, in this extravaganza of knowledge, to quench your academic thirst.

Preface

Dear Delegates,

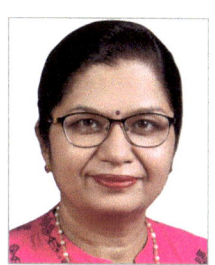

It is a pleasure to welcome you to Indore for AICOG 2022. The endoscopy workshop aims to teach a variety of surgical steps and skills required for day-to-day gynecological surgeries. After attending the workshop, the delegates should have learnt basic principles of endoscopy, relevant anatomy, various surgical approaches, pre- and postoperative management and various intraoperative tips and tricks. The workshop will feature interaction with the faculties as they perform surgeries live and also discussion mediated by a panel of experts.

This handout covers the basics and principles of gynecological endoscopic surgery, a good knowledge of which will help in understanding the techniques better and help in streamlining your surgical practices and avoid complications.

Wish you all happy learning!

Sumitra Yadav
Workshop Co-ordinator

Acknowledgments

We would like to acknowledge all the authors for sparing their invaluable time and intellectual skills towards the contribution of the chapters of this manual. We are also thankful to them for their prompt response in submission of the manuscript for the chapters of this manual.

We are also thankful to FOGSI team and the organizing team of AICOG 2022 for providing us the opportunity to contribute towards spreading the knowledge through this academic venture.

Contents

1. **Ergonomics in Gynecological Laparoscopy** 1
   Dhaval Baxi, Asha Baxi

2. **Energy Sources in Laparoscopy** 7
   Manjula Anagani, R Sindura Ganga, Swathi HV

3. **Safe Abdominal Port Entry Techniques in Laparoscopic Gynecologic Surgery** 14
   Vivek Salunke

4. **Diagnostic Laparoscopy** 21
   Yashodhan Deka

5. **Laparoscopic Anatomy of the Pelvis** 24
   Damodar Rao

6. **Diagnostic Hysteroscopy** 34
   Anshu Baser, Archana Baser

7. **Complications in Laparoscopy** 42
   B Ramesh, Jasmine S Abraham

8. **Complications in Hysteroscopy** 46
   S Krishnakumar, Aditi Abhade

9. **Sterilization and Disinfection in Endoscopy** 55
   Subash Mallya

10. **Myoma Specimen Retrieval Methods** 60
    Pandit Palaskar

CHAPTER 1

Ergonomics in Gynecological Laparoscopy

Dhaval Baxi, Asha Baxi

INTRODUCTION

Laparoscopic surgery in gynecology is mainstream and widely practiced. While this brings many benefits to the patient, injury to the surgeon is often under-reported. Careful theater layout and correct instruments minimize the risk to the surgeon. Ergonomics is the science of making the setting and surroundings favorable for the laparoscopic surgeon.

FACTORS AFFECTING THE SURGEON

Posture

A bent neck and back and a twisted torso tend to characterize the posture of a surgeon during open surgery, while laparoscopic procedures are characterized by a straight but twisted neck and a straight back. The poor ergonomic posture adopted by surgeons during both kinds of procedures can result in discomfort and, ultimately, injury. In addition, during laparoscopic surgery the upper limbs are often held in an excessive excursion/abduction in order to handle the long laparoscopic instruments, which pose additional musculoskeletal stresses compared with the equivalent open surgical procedure. The upright posture adopted during such procedures seems to be accompanied by substantially less body movement and weight shifting than during open surgery, allowing the build-up of lactic acid within the muscles, resulting in both pain and fatigue.

Footwear

Traditionally, surgeons wore clogs, footwear that has a nonflexible sole, whereas more recently most surgeons prefer footwear with a flexible sole. Placement of a gel mat under the surgeon's feet helps reduce musculoskeletal pain in the back, knees and feet during surgery which in return leads to less fatigue and fewer errors.

Age

Prevalence of backache among gynecologists increases with age, rising from a rate of 60% below the age of 40 years to 80% between 40 and 60 years of age.

Duration of Surgery and Stress Factors

The duration of the surgical procedure also appears to play a role in the prevalence of musculoskeletal symptoms among surgeons, with Cuschieri describing a "surgical fatigue syndrome" that occurred after 4 hours of laparoscopic surgery. The lack of three-dimensional vision, the fulcrum effect of instruments, having only 4 degrees of freedom of movement and the diminished tactile feedback encountered with laparoscopic surgery all affect the efficiency of the surgeon and hence operating time, which is inevitably increased compared with the equivalent open procedure.

Gender

In their study, Dolan and Martin reported that backache occurred more commonly in male (75.6%) than female (62.1%) gynecologists. This contrasts with the report by Stomberg et al. who found that female laparoscopic surgeons and gynecologists were more likely to experience musculoskeletal disorders than males despite being younger and having worked fewer years than their male counterparts. Although Park et al. found no differences in the prevalence of musculoskeletal symptoms between the sexes, they noted that male laparoscopic surgeons were more likely to suffer symptoms of the lower limbs while female surgeons reported more symptoms in the upper limbs.

OPTIMIZING THE ENVIRONMENT

Operating Table Height and Design

Working surface height relative to that of the subject performing manual work determines the upper extremity effort and the potential for musculoskeletal injury. Discomfort and surgical task difficulty are lowest when the handles of the instruments were positioned at the elbow height of the surgeon. In order to maintain instruments at elbow height, the ergonomic operating surface height should lie between 70 and 80% of the surgeon's ground to elbow distance, usually 650–1000 mm. Most current operating tables cannot be lowered enough to satisfy these ergonomic guidelines, thus changing the relation between the height of the surgeon's hands and the desirable height of the operating table. It is not uncommon for the surgeon to employ a step or platform to improve their ergonomic position but this should be large enough so that the surgeon can maintain their balance especially when using foot diathermy controls.

Design of the operating table is also important for laparoscopy of the pelvis. Operating in the pelvis often requires a steep Trendelenburg position to facilitate mobilization of the small bowel from the pelvis into the abdomen. In order to maintain the optimum operating table height in relation with the surgeon, one should position the patient in such a way that the patients' pelvis lies as close to the pillar of the operating table as possible. This will ensure that the pelvis does not rise when Trendelenburg position is given.

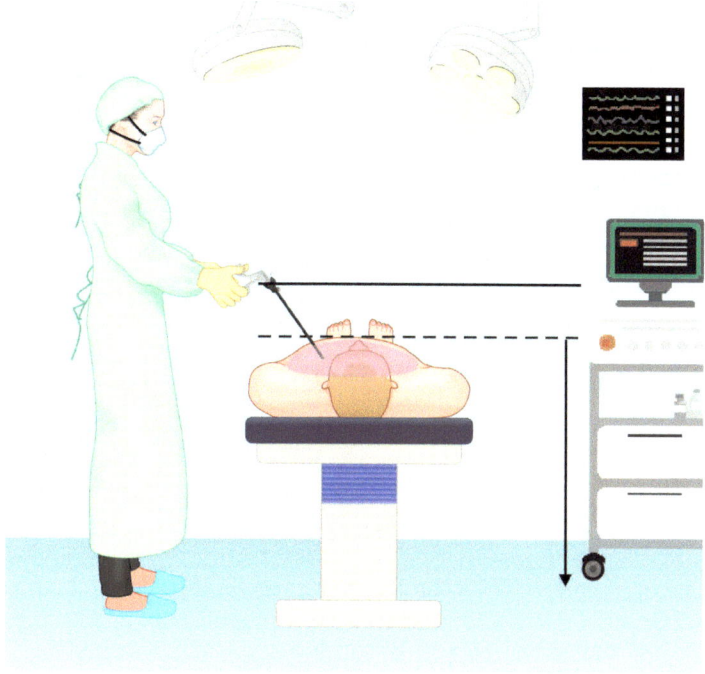

Fig.1: Operating table height and design.

Vaginal manipulation plays a key role in gynecological endoscopy. To facilitate the vaginal speculum placement and manipulation table manufacturers provide a C-shaped cut on the mattress of the operating table. The C-cut should be as close to the pillar as possible to ensure that the patient can be positioned close to the pillar of the operating table to maintain the optimum operating height **(Fig. 1)**.

Camera Systems

Initially endoscopic surgery was traditionally performed without using a camera. This lead to awkward postures of the surgeon and also restricting the use of one hand to hold the camera. It also restricted the ability of the assistant to help in surgery. With the advent of video laparoscopy there was an improvement in the posture of the surgeon. Improving quality in camera systems has increased the comfort of the surgeon with new 3D camera systems allowing depth perception and more accurate movements which helps reduce surgical fatigue.

Monitor Position

The position and height of the monitor will also impact on the degree of rotation or extension/flexion of the neck during laparoscopic surgery. In

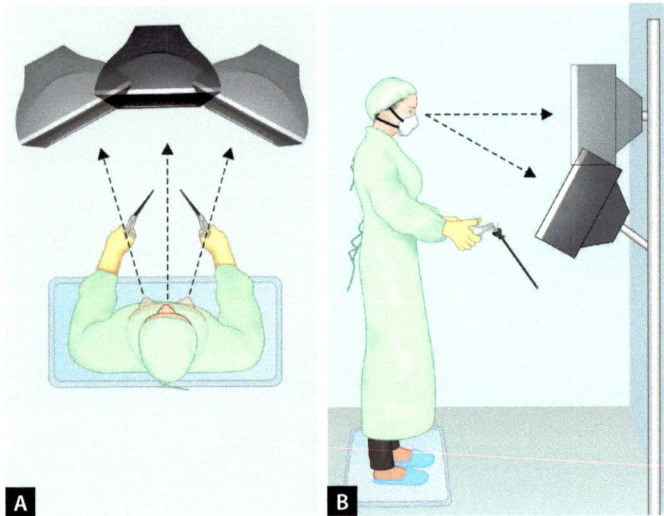

Figs. 2A and B: Monitor position.

many theaters, there is only one screen at the bottom of the bed, which necessitates axial rotation of the spine for the surgeon to see it. This will cause fatigue and muscle strain, especially during prolonged complex cases. Task performance is best when the screen is placed directly in front of the surgeon, in line with his or her forearm-motor axis.

The ideal height for the middle of the monitor is 5–9° below the horizontal plane of the eye or 20 cm below the height of the surgeon.

Distance of the monitor should also be ideal which is between 3 and 9 times the diagonal distance of the monitor. If a monitor is placed too far it may lead to excessive accommodation, convergence and staring and when placed too close it may lead to continuous and prolonged contraction of the extraocular and ciliary muscles which can lead to eye strain. The maximum distance can vary with the size of the monitor but the minimum distance should be at least 3 feet **(Figs. 2A and B)**.

Trocar Placement

Placement of trocars is crucial to smooth operating experience. Incorrect port placement can lead to imprecise movements leading to prolongation of the surgical time and musculoskeletal problems. Some surgeons prefer to place the trocars in a triangulation pattern while others in a sectorization fashion. The aim is to allow smooth manipulation of instruments and adequate laparoscopic visualization. The target organ should be around 15–20 cm away from the central trocar with a minimum distance of 10 cm. The remaining trocars should be placed around the central trocar allowing the instruments to work at a 60–90° angle.

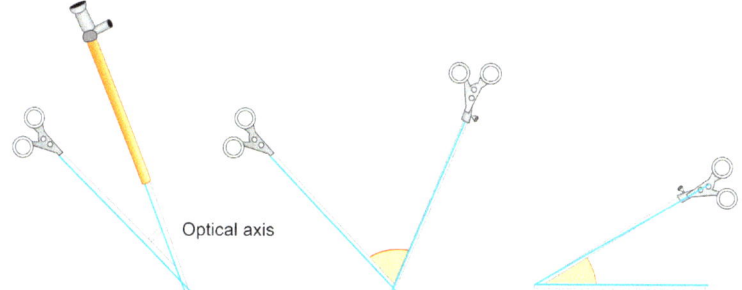

Fig. 3: Manipulation angles of instruments

Manipulation Angles of Instruments

- Optimal manipulation, elevation and azimuth angles are required for maximal laparoscopic task performance.
- Azimuth angle is the angle between the instrument and the optical axis of the endoscope.
- Manipulation angle is the angle between two instruments.
- Elevation angle is the angle between the instrument and the horizontal plane.
- The ideal manipulation angle should be between 45° and 60° and the azimuth and elevation angle should be the same for optimal performance **(Fig. 3)**.

Instrument-related Challenges

Laparoscopic instruments have limited freedom of movement compared to open surgeries. There are only 4 degrees of movement (in and out, left and right, rotation, and up and down) compared to full 360° hand movement. Articulation at the tip enhances tool's degrees of freedom. This in turn will provide a more comfortable mechanism for the surgeon thus increasing patient safety by reducing surgeon's fatigue which is the case with robotic surgery.

Handles of laparoscopic instruments are usually of a single size and a study demonstrated that surgeons with a glove size less than 6.5 had a difficulty in operating those instruments. Getting different handle sizes depending on the glove size may improve ease of instrument use. Using a shorter instrument shaft length (250 mm) also reduces the execution time of a task compared to longer shaft (330 mm) instruments.

Arm Support

Support of the elbow and shoulder has been shown to reduce fatigue and improve surgical accuracy in both microsurgery and neurosurgery. In addition, a study in 2005 reported that support of the shoulder, elbow and wrist significantly improved the accuracy of laparoscopic manipulations by the laparoscopic surgeon. Jafri et al. reported that armrests not only reduced the surgical error rate from 42.3 to 35% during simulated minimal access surgery, but also reduced oxygen consumption and resulted in improved operator comfort levels.

Physical Fitness

Endurance training of trunk muscles has shown to reduce fatigue of the operating surgeon.

Foot Pedals

Use of multiple foot pedals in laparoscopy to for activation of various energy sources, recording devices or morcellators, etc., require the surgeon to keep his foot in dorsiflexion. This position may impact the stability of the surgeon and also put strain on the surgeons' posture by putting more weight on the opposite leg. It can also result in anterior compartment pain in the leg controlling the foot pedals. Manufacturers have now developed instruments with hand controls and multiple functions but sometimes these may be difficult to control with one hand. Manufacturers should also explore at designing a more ergonomic system for control of the foot pedals which may help in reduction in surgeon fatigue.

Energy Sources

Use of advanced energy sources with combined coagulation and cutting features have helped in reducing the surgical time and also increased the safety margin. These advancements lead to reduction in hand movements and therefore help in reducing fatigue of the surgeon. Ultrasonic energy devices also have a cavitation feature which facilitates dissection of potential spaces.

■ CONCLUSION

Operating ergonomics is important for increasing operating efficiency and comfort of the surgeon which directly translates to better surgical performance and outcome. Careful attention should be paid towards the equipment design when setting up or upgrading an endoscopy unit. Ergonomics training should be developed and implemented in order to protect surgeons from preventable, potentially career-altering injuries.

■ SUGGESTED READING

1. Catanzarite T, Tan-Kim J, Menefee SA. Ergonomics in gynecologic surgery. Curr Opin Obstet Gynecol. 2018 Dec;30(6):432-440. doi: 10.1097/GCO.0000000000000502. PMID: 30299323.
2. Jhamb B. Lights, Camera, Action and ... Ergonomics in Gynecology Laparoscopy. Pan Asian J Obs Gyn. 2018;1(1):12-17.
3. Quinn D, Moohan J. Optimal laparoscopic ergonomics in gynaecology. The Obstetrician & Gynaecologist. 2015;17:77-82.

CHAPTER 2: Energy Sources in Laparoscopy

Manjula Anagani, R Sindura Ganga, Swathi HV

Minimally invasive surgery has undergone many advances over the recent years. Monopolar electrosurgery, bipolar electrosurgery, advanced bipolar devices, ultrasonic energy and various types of lasers are some of the technologies used nowadays to facilitate surgeons' tasks during laparoscopic operations.

A lack of basic knowledge or ignorance of principles of electrosurgery and equipment results in injuries during laparoscopic electrosurgery leading to significant morbidity and mortality and medicolegal actions. It is important though that surgeons have an understanding of the biophysics of these technologies in order to understand their limitations and potential dangers and to utilize the most appropriate energy source in the appropriate clinical setting to minimize the risk of a potential complication. Our skills will improve over time, thus enhancing patient satisfaction rates. Technique and technology are the two tiers of the vehicle called surgery which are both essential for the safe and successful outcomes.

The origin of electrosurgery dates back to 1877, when P Bozzini described the construction of a device for electrocauterization. In 1893, the high-frequency electric current was first used for treatment purposes. Several decades later in 1928, Bovie organized a production of electrosurgical equipment and described three different effects of this energy type: desiccation, dissection, and coagulation, which led to the establishment of fundamentals in modern electrosurgery and converted diagnostic laparoscopy into operative.

Hemostasis is basic in all surgical procedures. Traditional methods of staples and clips have gradually been abandoned due to cost, difficulty with repeated applications, and problems of displacement. Standard energy devices monopolar and bipolar coagulation are currently widely used due to their inexpensive nature and reusability. Also, the new vessel sealing technologies are so successful that they have largely made the need for laparoscopic suturing of vascular pedicles redundant. However, this involves high instrument cost, thermal spread, and sticking and charring of tissues.

PRINCIPLES OF ELECTROSURGERY

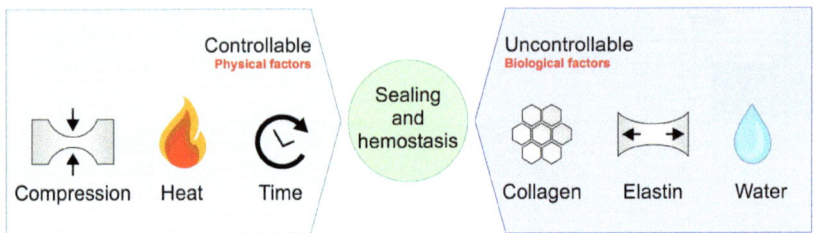

Other factors that may influence the tissue effect are size and shape of electrode, time of electric application, tissue resistance and whether the electrode touches or not the tissue.

TISSUE EFFECTS OF ELECTROSURGERY

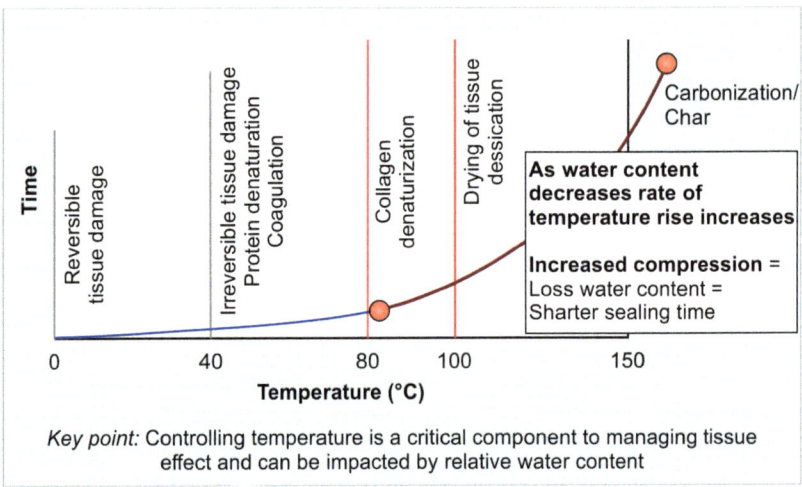

Key point: Controlling temperature is a critical component to managing tissue effect and can be impacted by relative water content

Approximate degree of heat	Thermal damage caused
<40°C	Reversible cell damage, depending on the duration of exposure
>40°C	Irreversible cell damage (denaturation)
>80°C	Coagulation, collagens are converted to glucose
>100°C	• Phase transition from liquid to vapor of intracellular and extracellular water • Tissue rapidly dries out (desiccation)
>150°C	Carbonization medical pathologic burns of 4th degree

Cutting requires the generation of sparks of brief duration between the electrode and the tissue. The heat from these sparks is transferred to the tissue producing cutting. As electrons in the form of sparks bombard cells, the energy transferred to them increases the temperature in a cell. As the temperature in the cell continues to rapidly increase, the pressure and volume of gases in the cell must also increase (PV = nrT). As a result, a temperature is reached at which the cell explodes. The best wave for cutting is a nonmodulated pure sine wave because current is delivered to the tissue almost 100% of the time the electrosurgical delivery device is activated.

Cutting achieved by an electrosurgical blade or spatula that is in contact with the tissue as a result of tissue heating and mechanical cleavage of the tissue.

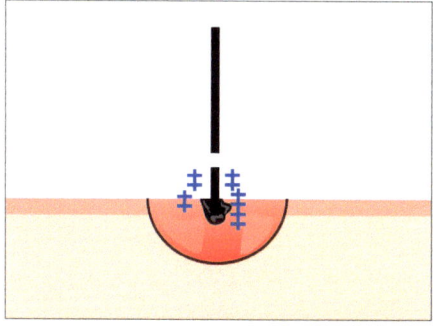

Fulguration or superficial coagulation also requires that there be no contact between the electrosurgical delivery device and the tissue. In contrast to cutting, fulguration requires a high enough voltage to produce sparks but a low power to produce coagulation rather than cutting. This is achieved by intermittent short bursts of high voltage. In effect, the temperature of the cell increases when it is hit by sparks but then returns towards normal as there is a prolonged period without any electron bombardment. The fulguration current is delivered via the coagulation switch of the electrosurgical generator.

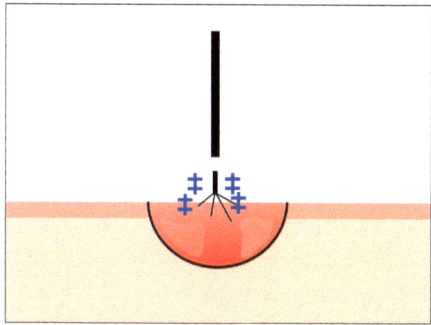

Desiccation or deep coagulation is the process by which the tissue is heated and the water in the cell boils to steam, resulting in a drying out of the cell. Desiccation can be achieved with either the cutting or the coagulation current by contact of the electrosurgical device with the tissue because no sparks are generated. Therefore, desiccation is a low power coagulation without sparking and it is the most common electrosurgical effect used by surgeons.

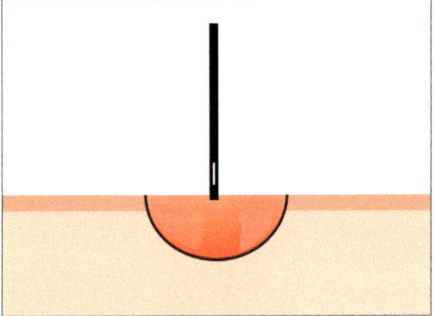

TYPES OF LAPAROSCOPIC ENERGY SOURCES AND THEIR TISSUE EFFECTS

Energy source	Tissue effects
Monopolar electrosurgery	Vaporization, fulguration, desiccation, coaptation
Conventional bipolar electrosurgery	Desiccation, coaptation
Advanced bipolar electrosurgery	Desiccation, coaptation, blade tissue transection
Ultrasonic technology	Desiccation, coaptation, mechanical tissue transection

The basic principle of electrosurgery is that the circuit must be completed.

The 3 basic components of electrosurgery:
1. Electrosurgical generator
2. Active electrode
3. Passive electrode

The electrosurgical generator converts the electric current from the low frequency electrical power outlets (60 Hz) to a high frequency electric current (>100 kHz), so it can not cause nerve and muscle stimulation.

Modern generators are isolated systems in which the therapeutic current is isolated from the power current by a transformer. The therapeutic current must return to the electrosurgical unit itself to complete the circuit. The result is virtually elimination of current diversion and alternate site burns.

Minimally invasive surgery has undergone significant advances and has changed the way operations are performed in the field of gynecology and its subspecialties.

Monopolar Electrosurgery

Current flows from active electrode (needle, hook, spatula or ball) → tissue and rest of the body → exits through passive (return) → electrode electrosurgical generator. Here, patient is a part of the circuit. Return electrode should be applied over a wide area such as muscle (good conducting surface) and avoid bony prominences.

Bipolar Electrosurgery

Involves only small amount of tissue in the circuits. Active and passive electrodes are close to each other and patient is not a part of the circuit. Desiccation is limited to the tissue in between, hence superior to monopolar. Vaporization and fulguration are inefficient and in order to transect the desiccated tissue we need to change instruments inducing this way the operating time.

Advanced Bipolar Devices (Ligasure, Enseal, etc.)

In addition to the features of conventional bipolar electrosurgery, advanced bipolar energy sources are revolutionary in several ways.
- Lateral thermal damage is reduced and tissue charring is minimized by, ESU—a computer—controlled tissue feedback system, where tissue impedance is monitored to maintain the lowest possible power setting to achieve the desired tissue effect, at which time an audio signal alerts the surgeon that the endpoint has been reached.
- US Food and Drug Administration (FDA) approved to seal vessels up to 7 mm in diameter owing to technological advances such as: tissue impedance monitoring up to 4000 times per second (LigaSure); temperature-sensitive material in the device jaws that optimizes tissue temperatures at ~100°C (EnSeal); and jaw design that optimizes mechanical compression to the vascular pedicle (LigaSure, EnSeal).

Hence, the decision to use a particular bipolar device may come down to dissection capability versus instrument traffic. Although advanced bipolar energy sources are relatively expensive, they are generally available in most hospitals.

Ultrasonic Devices (Harmonic Ace, Sonicision)

The principle of ultrasonic energy is conversion of electrical energy into mechanical and thermal energy via ultrasonic vibrations to achieve tissue transection and vessel sealing. In addition to mechanical friction, *"cavitation effect"* may facilitate transection. Cavitation is the phenomenon that occurs during tissue vaporization and the steam released from vaporized cells expands existing tissue planes, assisting dissection.

Advantages of ultrasonic devices include less instrument traffic, owing to the combination of vessel-sealing and tissue cutting, and less smoke generation.

Hybrid Devices (Thunderbeat, Ligasure Advance)

Thunderbeat is the first device to integrate both ultrasonically generated frictional heat energy and advanced bipolar energy in one instrument. It can rapidly cut and precisely dissect tissue while advanced bipolar technology provides vessel sealing up to 7 mm diameter with minimal thermal spread. The generator has level 1 for cutting and sealing while level 3 for sealing mode. Ligasure Advance has recently been developed that combine several energy source technologies.

Laser (Light Amplification by Stimulated Emission of Radiation)

There are a number of different types of lasers: CO_2, argon, Nd:YAG, KTP-532 with different properties. The accuracy of targeting tissues and lack of lateral thermal spread.

In gynecology they are mainly used for endometriosis ablation as they are not absorbed by unpigmented tissues and thus abnormal tissues are preferably coagulated.

COMPLICATIONS OF ENERGY SOURCES IN LAPAROSCOPY

The rate of electrosurgical complications during delivery of energy to the surgical site is estimated to be 25.6% (70/273) and is the second most common laparoscopic complication after a misplacement of trocar or Veress needle.

Injuries during laparoscopic electrosurgical procedures are similar to those during laparotomy and can be attributed to misidentification of anatomic structures, mechanical trauma, or electrothermal injuries.

The mechanism of injuries can be in the form of:
- Direct damage from mistaken targeting or unintended activation.
- A stray current arising from defective insulation can injure the bowel or blood vessels
- *Direct coupling*: Occurs when the active electrode is accidentally activated or is in close proximity to another metal instrument within the pelvic cavity.
- *Capacitive coupling*: Occurs when the electric current is transferred from one conductor (the active electrode), through intact insulation, into adjacent conductive materials (e.g., bowel) without direct contact.
- If the return electrode is not completely in contact with the patient's skin, or is not able to disperse the current safely, then the exiting current can lead to an unintended burn.

- Delayed manifestation of bladder injury may result in vesicovaginal fistula, which requires repetitive repair if the first salvage procedure fails.

Because electrosurgical complications are an inevitable reality of laparoscopy, it is important to have a systematic awareness of the types of complications, know how to respond appropriately, and know how to communicate and deal with complications. To achieve electrosurgical safety and prevent potential electrosurgical injury, it is crucial to not understand the biophysics of electrosurgery, characteristics of the equipment used, desired tissue effects, types of injury, and the possible clinical manifestations, and also master laparoscopic surgical dexterity.

CONCLUSION

Efficiency, safety, and efficacy are inextricably linked to the thoughtful orchestration of all of these elements. When experience and judgment are coupled with fundamental knowledge, then science becomes art in the hands of the laparoscopic surgeon.

We should constantly review our techniques and instrumentation to maximize patient safety.

FINAL THOUGHTS

Complications happen, even in the very best of hands. None of us are immune to complications. The strategies that we currently follow, based on 15 years of gynec endoscopic experience and based on complications suffered by others' and my own patients have been suggested.

Hence, it is likely that the surgeon will rely on two or more laparoscopic energy sources (or hybrid instruments incorporating multiple technologies) depending on the cost and availability of the devices (and their proprietary ESUs), personal preference and experience, the surgical procedure to be performed, and the presence or absence of significant pathology in the surgical field.

I realize that many suggestions remain controversial, and well respected colleagues will disagree with many of them. However, I hope that you will consider incorporating at least some of these strategies in your practice. I want you to have a long, successful, and happy career in gynecologic surgery.

CHAPTER 3

Safe Abdominal Port Entry Techniques in Laparoscopic Gynecologic Surgery

Vivek Salunke

INTRODUCTION

Laparoscopy has gradually become popular in gynecological practices due to its many benefits and has less surgical complications compared to laparotomy such as pain and hospitalization. Complications related to gynecological laparoscopy are relatively rare but mostly related with abdominal port entry. It is a challenging procedure in laparoscopy because of its serious complications such as gastrointestinal tract and major blood vessel injuries that account for 50% cases prior to the commencement of the intended surgery. Most injuries are caused by the insertion of the primary umbilical trocar, so it is important to learn the safe techniques in creating pneumoperitoneum in gynecologic laparoscopy.

The main abdominal access techniques used in laparoscopic surgery include:
1. Classic or closed entry
2. Open (Hasson) technique
3. Direct trocar insertion without prior pneumoperitoneum

CLOSED ENTRY (CLASSIC) LAPAROSCOPY

The classic, or closed entry, laparoscopic technique requires cutting of the abdominal skin with a scalpel, insufflation of air or gas into the abdomen (establishment of pneumoperitoneum), and insertion of a sharp trocar/cannula system into the abdomen. Following removal of the sharp trocar, the abdominal cavity is examined by an illuminated telescope through the cannula.

Veress Needle Insertion Sites (Fig. 1)

1. *Umbilical point:* Here there is risk of injury to abdominal viscera, inferior vena cava (IVC) and abdominal aorta.
2. *Palmer's point* is most preferred site for port entry. It lies in left upper quadrant 3 cm below left subcostal margin in mid-clavicular line and is preferred in obese, very thin females or previously operated for abdominal surgeries. In Palmer's point, one must be careful of inflated stomach so must deflate it using nasogastric tube, in cases of hepatosplenomegaly,

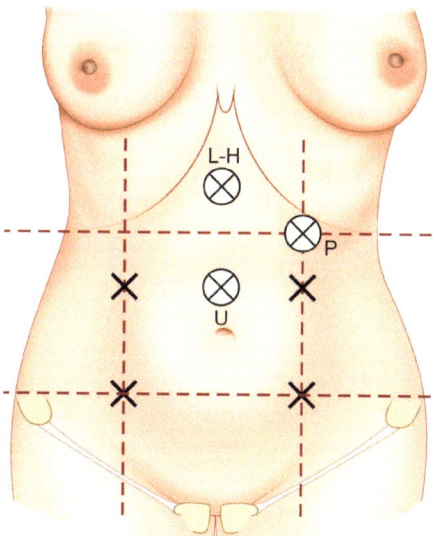

Fig. 1: The access points for abdominal entry in laparoscopic surgery. (L-H = Lee-Huang point; P = Palmer's point; U = umbilical point)

previous gastric or splenic surgery and careful of splenic flexure of colon in case of tuberculosis.

3. *Jain point* lies in the left paraumbilical region in a straight line of 10–13 cm depending on patient's body mass index (BMI) and body type drawn vertically upward from a point of 2.5 cm medial and 1 cm above anterior-superior iliac spine. It avoids sudden catastrophic injury to major retroperitoneal vessels, viscera, adhesions and bowel.
4. *Lee-Huang point* lies at the middle upper abdomen centrally between the xiphoid process and the umbilicus and preferred in large pelvic pathology like fibroids, gynecological malignancy or failed Palmer's or umbilical approach, umbilical hernia.
5. *Latif's point* is in the right angle between the xiphoid process and the right costal margin but there is risk of injury to liver and must be avoided in previous right upper abdominal operated or mass cases.
6. *Transuterine Veress CO_2 insufflation:* Using a long Veress needle, pneumoperitoneum has been established through the fundus of the uterus transvaginally. This technique has been especially helpful in obese women.
7. *Trans cul-de-sac CO_2 insufflation:* The posterior vaginal fornix has been reported as another site through which to establish pneumoperitoneum especially in obese women.
8. *Ninth or tenth intercostal space CO_2 insufflation:* If the parietal peritoneum is adhered to the undersurface of the ribs at the costal margin, Veress needle

can be inserted through the ninth or tenth intercostal space at the anterior axillary line along the superior surface of the lower rib to avoid injury to the underlying neurovascular bundle. Following pneumoperitoneum, established at 20-25 mm Hg pressure, 5 mm laparoscopes are introduced at Palmer's point for inspection, followed by additional trocars, inserted under direct vision, to facilitate the required surgery and/or perform adhesiolysis when indicated.

Angle of Veress Needle Insertion

The position of the umbilicus was found, on average, 0.4 cm, 2.4 cm, and 2.9 cm caudally to the aortic bifurcation in normal weight (BMI <25 kg/m^2), overweight (BMI 25-30 kg/m^2), and obese (BMI >30 kg/m^2) women, respectively. Therefore, the angle of the Veress needle insertion should vary accordingly from 45° in non-obese women to 90° in very obese women.

Veress Needle Safety Tests

- The double click sound of the Veress needle
- The aspiration test
- The hanging drop of saline test
- The "hiss" sound test
- The syringe test

Veress Needle Modifications

To reduce entry-related injuries several instruments have been introduced like—shielded disposable trocars, optical Veress needle, optical trocars, radially expanding trocars, and a trocarless reusable, visual access cannula.
- *Pressure-sensor-equipped Veress needle:* A modified pressure-sensor-equipped Veress needle to provide the surgeon immediate feedback the moment the tip enters the peritoneal cavity has been described.
- *Optical Veress needle (minilaparoscopy):* The Veress needle has been modified to a 2.1 mm diameter and cannula 10.5 cm long to allow insertion of a thin zero degree, semirigid fiberoptic minilaparoscope. During insertion of the assembled unit (Veress cannula and telescope) the surgeon observes a cascade of monitor color sequences that represent different abdominal wall layers: subcutaneous fat appears yellow, fascia white, anterior rectus muscle red, and peritoneum translucent or shiny bright.

Veress Intraperitoneal (VIP) Pressure

Several investigators have reported initial intraperitoneal insufflation pressures <10 mm Hg indicating correct Veress needle placement. Adequate pneumoperitoneum traditionally has been defined by an arbitrary volume of 1 L to 4 L of CO_2 or an arbitrary intraperitoneal pressure of 10–15 mm Hg.

High Pressure Entry (The HIP Entry)

The pressure technique has been adopted by many surgeons worldwide, but the appropriate volume to establish an appropriate intra-abdominal pressure remains controversial. Final pressures up to 10 mm Hg, 15 mm Hg, 14–18 mm Hg, 20 mm Hg, and even 25–30 mm have been advocated.

The rationale for the higher pressure entry technique is that it produces greater splinting of the anterior abdominal wall and a deeper intra-abdominal CO_2 bubble than the traditional volume-limited pneumoperitoneum of 2–4 L.

It has been determined that trocar insertion requires 4–6 kg of force, and shielded disposable trocars require half the force of reusable trocars.

It has been demonstrated that the use of transient high-pressure pneumoperitoneum causes minor hemodynamic alterations of no clinical significance.

■ OPEN LAPAROSCOPIC ENTRY OR HASSON TECHNIQUE

Hasson first described the open entry technique in 1971. The suggested benefits are prevention of gas embolism, of preperitoneal insufflation, and possibly of visceral and major vascular injury.

The technique involves using a cannula fitted with a cone-shaped sleeve, a blunt obturator, and possibly a second sleeve to which stay sutures can be attached. A small incision is made transversely or longitudinally at the umbilicus. The cannula is inserted into the peritoneal cavity with the blunt obturator in place. Sutures are placed on either side of the cannula in the fascia and attached to the cannula or purse-stringed around the cannula to seal the abdominal wall incision to the cone-shaped sleeve. The laparoscope is then introduced and insufflation is commenced.

The open technique is favored by general surgeons and considered by some to be indicated in patients with previous abdominal surgery, especially those with longitudinal abdominal wall incisions.

Most common of the major complications associated with access were bowel injuries. The risk of bowel injury was higher with the open technique than with closed technique, technique (0.09%).

■ DIRECT TROCAR ENTRY

The suggested advantages of this method of entry are the avoidance of complications related to the use of the Veress needle: failed pneumoperitoneum, preperitoneal insufflation, intestinal insufflation, or the more serious CO_2 embolism.

Laparoscopic entry is initiated with only one blind step (trocar) instead of three (Veress needle, insufflation, trocar). The direct entry method is faster than any other method of entry however, it is the least performed laparoscopic technique in clinical practice today.

The technique begins with an infra-umbilical skin incision wide enough to accommodate the diameter of a sharp trocar/cannula system. The anterior abdominal wall must be adequately elevated by hand, and the trocar is inserted directly into the cavity, aiming towards the pelvic hollow. On removal of the sharp trocar, the laparoscope is inserted to confirm the presence of omentum or bowel in the visual field. A history of abdominal surgery was not associated with an increased risk of complications.

Sharp trocars are recommended for a direct insertion technique.

Direct insertion of the trocar is associated with less insufflation-related complications such as gas embolism, and it is a faster technique than the Veress needle technique.

Disposable-shielded Trocars

Disposable shielded "safety" trocars were introduced in 1984. These trocars are designed with a shield that partially retracts and exposes the sharp tip as it encounters resistance through the abdominal wall. As the shield enters the abdominal cavity, it springs forward and covers the sharp tip of the trocar. These trocars were intended to prevent the sharp tip from injuring intra-abdominal contents. Shielded trocars may be used in an effort to decrease entry injuries, however, there is no evidence that they result in fewer visceral and vascular injuries during laparoscopic access.

Radially Expanding Access System

Advantages of this system include elimination of sharp trocars, application of radial force, stabilization of the cannula's position (cannula does not slide in and out), avoidance of injury to abdominal wall vessels, and elimination of the need for suturing of fascial defects. Radially expanding trocars are not recommended as being superior to the traditional trocars. They do have blunt tips that may provide some protection from injuries, but the force required for entry is significantly greater than with disposable trocars.

Visual Entry Systems

Disposable Optical Trocars Optical/access trocars were introduced in 1949 and are popular among urologists. Two disposable visual entry systems are available that retain the conventional trocar and cannula push-through design: the Endopath Optiview optical trocar (Ethicon Endo-Surgery, Inc., Cincinnati, OH) and the VisiPort™ optical trocar (Tyco-United States Surgical, Norwalk, CT). These single-use visual trocars trade blind sharp trocars for a hollow trocar, in which a zero-degree laparoscope is loaded for the distal crystal tip to transmit real-time monitor images while transecting abdominal wall tissue layers.

Endopath Optiview Optical Trocar

This comprises a hollowed trocar and a cannula. When insufflation is complete, the Veress needle is withdrawn, and the subcutaneous fatty tissue is dissected off, using peanut sponges, to expose the white anterior rectus fascia. A 5-mm incision is then made with a scalpel to accommodate the visual trocar's pointed tip. The fascia is then divided between the stay sutures over a length of approximately 5 mm. During insertion, the stay sutures are pulled to lift the abdominal wall against the advancing trajectory and facilitate proper port site closure at the end of the operation. The cascade of generated entry images displayed on the monitor demonstrates level of penetration.

VisiPort™ Optical Trocars

The VisiPort™ optical trocar is a disposable visual entry instrument that comprises a hollow trocar and a cannula. When insufflation is complete, the Veress needle is withdrawn, and subcutaneous fatty tissue is dissected off, downward axial pressure is applied while activating the trigger. Then downward pressure is relieved, the trigger released, and the trocar tip position verified on the monitor again. This entry sequence is repeated until the peritoneal cavity is entered. The trigger is not fired until the exact anatomical position of the trocar tip is known. The push-through entry design requires significant perpendicular force to drive a trajectory across tissue planes with no means of avoiding trocar overshoot.

The VisiPort™ optical trocar comes in only one diameter and accommodates only a 10-mm laparoscope.

EndoTIP Visual Cannula

The endoscopic threaded imaging port, EndoTIP (Karl STORZ Endoscopy, Tuttlingen, Germany), is a reusable visual cannula system that allows real-time interactive port creation, when port-dynamics are archived, for recall and analysis.

The visual entry cannula system may represent an advantage over traditional trocars, as it allows a clear optical entry, but this advantage has not been fully explored. The visual entry cannula trocars have the advantage of minimizing the size of the entry wound and reducing the force necessary for insertion. Visual entry trocars are non-superior to other trocars since they do not avoid visceral and vascular injury.

In 2019, Cochrane review authors evaluated the benefits and risks of different laparoscopic entry techniques in gynecological and non-gynecological surgery. Systematic review authors included 57 randomized controlled trials with a total of 9865 individuals undergoing laparoscopy. There was insufficient evidence to show whether there were differences between groups in the rate of failed entry, vascular injury, or visceral injury, or in other major complications with the use of an open-entry technique in comparison to a closed-entry technique. Overall conclusion was that the evidence was insufficient to support the use of one laparoscopic entry technique over another. Researchers noted an advantage of direct trocar entry over Veress needle entry for failed entry. Most evidence was of very low quality; the main limitations were imprecision (due to small sample sizes and very low event rates) and risk of bias associated with poor reporting of study methods.

CONCLUSION

Many techniques have been introduced to eliminate laparoscopic entry complications; however, not a single technique has been proven to eliminate this complication. On comparing open and closed techniques, there is no difference in the incidence of visceral or vascular injury. Thus, to prevent and decrease complications of port entry, surgeons should continue to increase their knowledge of anatomy, their training, and their experience.

SUGGESTED READING

1. Ellison E, Zollinger RM, Jr (Eds.). Hasson open technique for laparoscopic access. Zollinger's Atlas of Surgical Operations, 10th edition. McGraw Hill. 2016. [online] Available from https://accesssurgery.mhmedical.com/content.aspx?bookid= 1755&sectionid=119128026 [Last accessed March, 2022]
2. Jain N, Sareen S, Kanawa S, Jain V, Gupta S, Mann S. Jain point: A new safe portal for laparoscopic entry in previous surgery cases. J Hum Reprod Sci. 2016;9(1):9-17.
3. Lee CL, Huang KG, Jain S, Wang CJ, Yen CF, Soong YK. A new portal for gynecologic laparoscopy. J Am Assoc Gynecol Laparosc. 2001 Feb 1;8(1):147-50.
4. Palmer R. Safety in laparoscopy. J Reprod Med. 1974;13:1-5.

CHAPTER 4

Diagnostic Laparoscopy

Yashodhan Deka

INTRODUCTION
- Laparoscopy is a surgical procedure that has been used widely in medicine over 30 years. Faster recovery rate, the minimizing of pain, hospitalization and better aesthetic results are some of the advantages which made laparoscopy very popular among patients and surgeons. Also some technical parameters such as the magnification offered by the endoscope during the procedure and the small risk of complications resulted to the wide use of laparoscopic surgery in gynecology.
- It consists of endoscopic viewing of the abdominal cavity by means of distension provided by artificial pneumoperitoneum.
- The first description of laparoscopy was by Ott and Kelling in 1901.

WHAT IS DIAGNOSTIC LAPAROSCOPY?
- It is a type of surgical procedure classified as minimally invasive procedure.
- Laparoscopy allows surgeon to gain access to the peritoneal cavity, without having to make large incisions.
- Laparoscopy has proved to be an important tool in the minimally invasive exploration of selected patients with chronic disorders whose diagnosis remained uncertain despite exploring the requisite laboratory and imaging investigations.

INDICATIONS
- Laparoscopy can be used to assist in diagnosing a wide range of conditions that develop in peritoneal cavity.
- Categories includes:
    - Gynecologic
    - Gastrointestinal
    - Urologic
    - Musculoskeletal
    - Surgical
    - Vascular

Gynecological Indications
- Infertility work up—ovulation study
  - Tubal patency
  - Endometriosis
  - Pelvic adhesions
- Acute pelvic lesions
  - Acute ectopic
  - Acute salpingitis
- Pelvic mass—fibroid
  - Ovarian cysts
- Follow-up of pelvic surgery—tuboplasty
  - Ovarian malignancy
  - Evaluation of endometriosis treatment
- Suspected Müllerian abnormalities
- Suspected uterine perforation
- To take biopsy

CONTRAINDICATIONS
- Severe cardiopulmonary diseases
- Generalized peritonitis
- Intestinal obstruction
- Significant hemoperitoneum
- Large pelvic tumor
- Pregnancy >16 weeks
- Obesity
- Extensive pelvic adhesions

ADVANTAGES
Compared to traditional open surgery:
- Decrease in wound size
- Decrease in wound pain
- Improved mobility
- Reduction in wound infection, dehiscence, bleeding, herniation.
- Reduced hospital stay.

COMPLICATIONS OF LAPAROSCOPIC SURGERIES
- Anesthetic complications
- Complications due to pneumoperitoneum
- Surgical complications. Injuries to viscus
- *Stomach:* Injury may occur with trocar or needle.
- Bowel injuries also may occur with trocar or Veress needle.
- *Bladder injury:* Injury caused by second puncture trocar usually.

- *Ureter:* May be injured in adnexal surgeries. Thermal injuries will result in ureteral narrowing and hydroureter.
- *Vessels injuries:* Large vessels may be injured by trocar or Veress needle. CO_2 peritoneum may tamponade a large vessel injury. Vessels most commonly injured are—epigastric vessels, ovarian vessels, uterine vessels.
- Diathermy-related injuries—due to inadvertent activation of the diathermy pedal, faulty insulations, direct coupling. Diathermal injuries causes thermal necrosis of organs, inadvertent organ ligation, unrecognized hemorrhage.
- Patients factors-related complications—obesity, ascites, organomegaly, coagulation disorder.
- Postoperative complications.

CONCLUSION

Laparoscopic gynecologic surgery has become most common place in today's gynecologic practice. As a method, it provides many benefits for the patient as a minimal invasive procedure, either it is performed as a purely diagnostic procedure or as a surgical treatment. It is considered the gold standard method for exploring infertility or chronic pelvic pain as the gynecologist can explore with direct view the pelvis and the whole peritoneal cavity without subjecting the patient to the extend trauma of laparotomy.

Today more and more classic gynecologic operations are being replaced by laparoscopy. Despite numerous advantages it provides, it should not be considered a panacea, as it remains surgical procedure and has the risks of complications as every other procedure.

CHAPTER 5

Laparoscopic Anatomy of the Pelvis

Damodar Rao

INTRODUCTION

Basic knowledge of the pelvic anatomy is necessary for safe, effective and efficient laparoscopic surgery. Advancements in the field of laparoscopy in the areas of vision and pneumoperitoneum have significantly improved our understanding of pelvic anatomy. New spaces and planes have emerged after the adoption of laparoscopy and nerve sparing gynecological surgeries. Basic anatomy of the pelvis namely the bladder, uterus, fallopian tubes, ovary and rectum remain unchanged but the anatomy surrounding these structures namely the vessels, avascular spaces and ureter require a great deal of attention.

ANTERIOR ABDOMINAL WALL

The layers of the anterior abdominal wall consist of the skin, subcutaneous layer, rectus sheath, transversalis fascia and peritoneum. The parietal peritoneum being the inner most surface has five elevations or folds raised by different structures which converge towards the umbilicus and hence are called the umbilical ligaments.
- Median umbilical ligament—formed by the urachus extends from the apex of the bladder to the umbilicus.
- The medial umbilical ligaments are formed by the obliterated umbilical arteries. They are lateral to the median umbilical ligament. When traced proximally they lead to internal iliac artery and uterine arteries which play an important landmark in surgeries with frozen pelvis.
- The lateral umbilical ligaments are formed by the peritoneum covering the inferior epigastric artery prior to their entry into the rectus sheath. Identification of these ligaments is useful during accessory port placements. The lie medial to the deep inguinal ring and hence help in classifying the hernias into direct or indirect inguinal hernia.

Overall, the umbilical ligaments serve as valuable laparoscopic landmarks during any surgery.

Laparoscopic Anatomy of the Pelvis

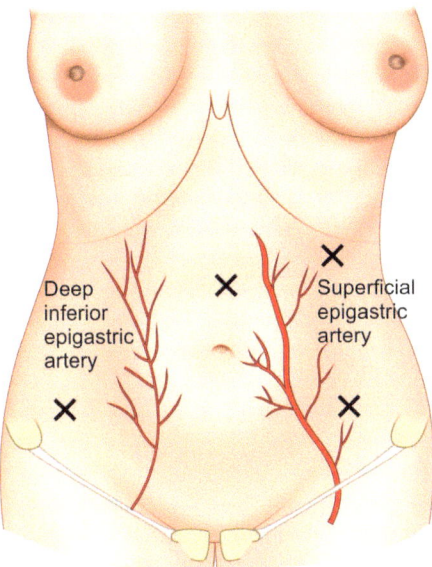

Fig. 1: Superficial epigastric artery and deep inferior epigastric artery.

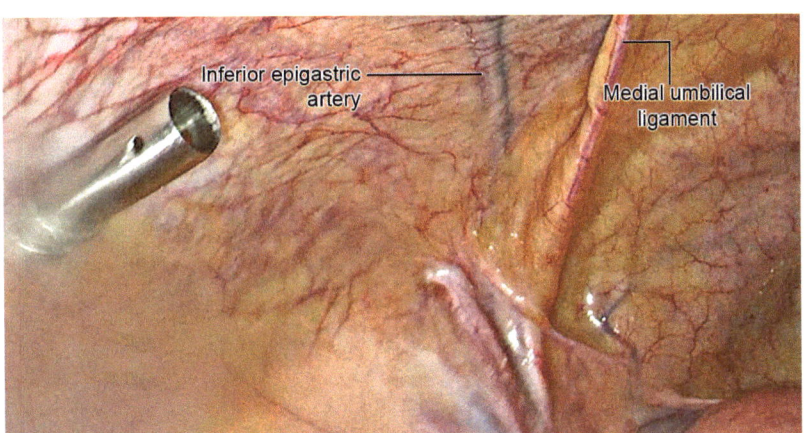

Fig. 2: Inferior epigastric artery.

ORGANS IN THE PELVIS

- Uterus
- Fallopian tubes
- Ovaries
- Bladder
- Rectum

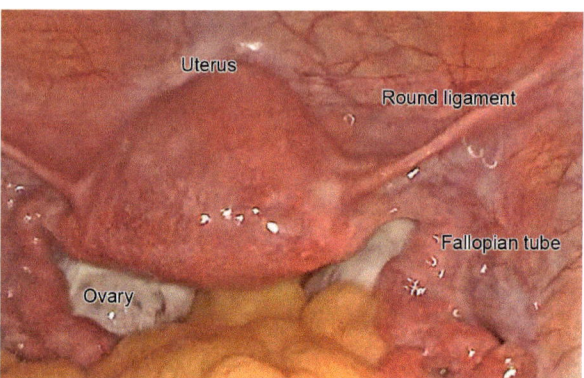

Fig. 3: Gross laparoscopic anatomy of the pelvis.

■ VASCULAR ANATOMY

The vascular system of the pelvis starts from the bifurcation of the abdominal aorta into the right and left common iliac artery at the level of sacral promontory. The sacral promontory forms an important landmark as the small bowel mesentery also crosses at this level thus separating the pelvic structures from upper abdominal organs.

The Inferior vena cava divides at a slightly lower level and to the left of the aorta.

The veins are always at a proximity to the arteries but lie posterior and hence lymphadenectomy can be easily achieved without injuring the veins.

The Common iliac artery further bifurcates into the external and the internal iliac artery.

External Iliac Artery and Vein

The external iliac vessels traverses along the iliopsoas muscle with the vein being posteromedial to the artery. Both are devoid of any branches in the pelvis facilitating easy pelvic lymph node dissection.

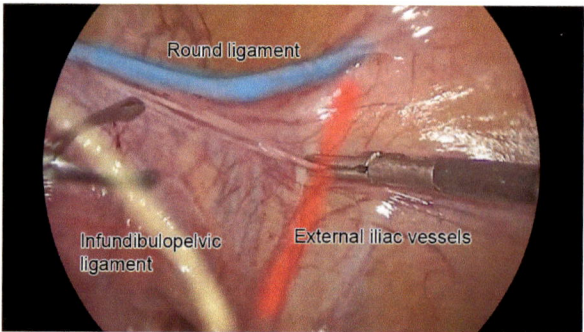

Fig. 4: Opening the pararectal space.

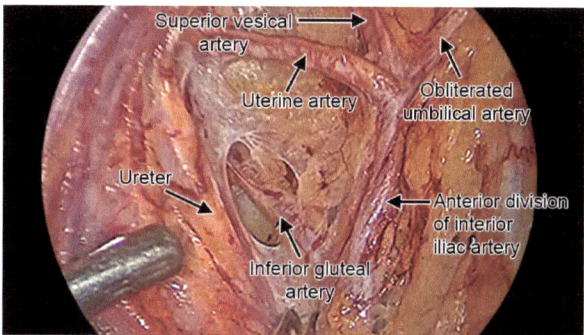

Fig. 5: Vascular anatomy of the right side of pelvis.

Internal Iliac Artery and Vein

The internal iliac courses downwards and at about 2–3 cm from its origin from the common iliac it divides into an anterior and posterior branch respectively. The anterior branch mainly supplies the pelvic organs through its various branches, namely the bladder, uterus, and the rectum. The posterior division pierces the presacral fascia to supply the gluteal region.

The first branch of the anterior division of the internal iliac artery is the uterine artery followed by the superior and inferior vesical arteries. The middle rectal artery which is a branch of the anterior division of the internal iliac is not visualized in almost 30% of the patients. The other branches include the obturator, the internal pudendal and inferior gluteal artery. Finally, the artery continues as the obliterated umbilical artery to the anterior abdominal wall.

The internal iliac vein is closely applied to the artery and hence one must be careful while dissecting the artery.

Uterine Artery and Vein

The first branch arising from the anterior division of the internal iliac artery is the uterine artery. It is tortuous and traverses a long distance before supplying the uterus. Hence, there is an adequate length available for ligation of the artery. On its way to the uterus, it crosses the ureter anteriorly and gives off a branch to the ureter. Once the pararectal space is opened, the first structure which crosses transversely is the uterine artery.

The artery enters the uterus at the level of internal os and it then divides into ascending and descending branches. The ascending branch forms the main supply of the uterus while the descending branch supplies the cervix and vagina.

The uterine vein runs underneath the ureter. The parasympathetic nerve fibers are closely applied to the vein and hence it is an important structure in nerve sparing surgery.

Ureter

The ureteric anatomy is the most important in any laparoscopic pelvic surgery. In adults, the length of the ureter from the renal pelvis to the trigone of the bladder is about 25–30 cm. The ureter is divided by the pelvic brim into the abdominal and pelvic segments. The ureter courses along psoas muscle at the level of the pelvic brim. At this level, it enters the pelvis crossing over the bifurcation of the common iliac artery from lateral to medial on the respective sides. It then courses down; just lateral to the sacrum up to the level of internal os. Here, it deviates medially, to lie next to the internal iliac artery and passes below the uterine artery. This is about 2 cm lateral to the internal os. From here, it passes through the ureteric tunnel and courses medially, lying anterior to the vaginal fornix, after which it enters the bladder.

The ureter gets its blood supply from the common iliac, internal iliac, uterine, and superior vesical vessels. Branches of these arteries form a vascular anastomosis along the length of the ureter.

The common sites of ureteric injury are—at the pelvic brim near the infundibulopelvic ligament, at the isthmus, pelvic sidewall, near the vaginal fornix.

It is important to trace the course of the ureter in cases of severe endometriosis and malignancies to prevent inadvertent injuries.

An attempt to achieve complete hemostasis thermal injury to ureter is the most common and one should be careful while using an energy source. It is important to know the extent of lateral spread of energy used during laparoscopic procedures, especially when dealing with structures near the ureters.

Nerves

The pelvic organs are supplied by the sympathetic nerves from T10-L2 and parasympathetic nerves from S2, S3 and S4. They together emerge to form the inferior hypogastric plexus which supply the uterus and the bladder. In nerve sparing radical hysterectomy, only the uterine fibers are divided and fibers innervating the bladder are preserved.

The other nerves are the genitofemoral nerve and the obturator nerve. The genitofemoral nerve lies along the lateral side of external iliac artery and should be protected during pelvic lymph node dissection.

The obturator nerve forms the inferior limit for the pelvic lymph node dissection.

Lymphatics

The pelvic lymph nodes play a crucial role in gynecologic oncology. The pelvic lymph nodes are the external iliac nodes along the external iliac artery and vein caudally up to the deep circumflex vein, the obturator nodes in the obturator fossa, the internal iliac nodes course along the hypogastric vessels.

Avascular Spaces

Avascular spaces are delineated by separating two independent fasciae and contain loose areolar tissue. Exposing these spaces early in the surgery avoids injury to vital structures like ureter, nerves and blood vessels.

Pelvic spaces are divided into lateral and median space.

Lateral spaces are:
- Paravesical space
- Pararectal space
- Yabuki space

Median spaces are:
- Space of Retzius
- Vesicovaginal/Vesicocervical
- Rectovaginal space
- Presacral space

Paravesical Space

Paravesical space is bounded by:
- Anteriorly—superior pubic ramus
- Posteriorly—uterine artery and vein
- Medially—bladder
- Laterally—obturator internus fascia and muscle, external iliac artery and vein.

The important contents of the space are the obliterated umbilical artery, obturator neurovascular bundle, accessory obturator artery, superior vesical artery, lymphatic tissue.

The obturator umbilical artery divides the space into lateral paravesical and medial paravesical space respectively. This space is of importance during radical hysterectomy for complete removal of uterus along with its attachments and for pelvic lymphadenectomy. The limit of dissection would be the obturator nerve. The medial paravesical space also forms an access point for bladder dissection in conditions of dense uterovesical adhesions seen in patients with history of previous cesarean section.

Pararectal Space

The space bounded on either side of the rectum forms the pararectal space.

It is bounded by:
- Ventrally—cardinal ligament
- Dorsally—sacrum and the presacral fascia
- Medially—rectum
- Laterally—internal iliac artery

The ureter being one of the important structures of the pararectal space, divides it into lateral Latzko space and the medial Okabayashi space.

The Latzko space dissection exposes the uterine artery origination from the internal iliac artery, hence it is important in various cases like radical hysterectomy, large myomas requiring temporary ligation of uterine artery, pelvic lymphadenectomy, adhesions due to previous pelvic surgeries.

The Okabayashi space is developed by incising and opening space between the posterior leaf of broad ligament and the ureter. The Okabayashi space is developed in cases where ureter mobilization is required, for bowel management and major ureter surgery in deeply infiltrative endometriosis.

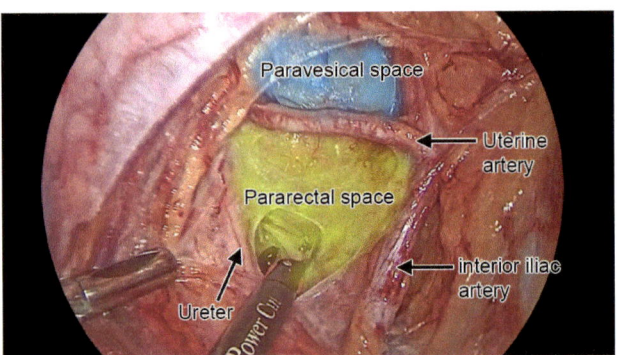

Fig. 6: Pararectal and paravesical space.

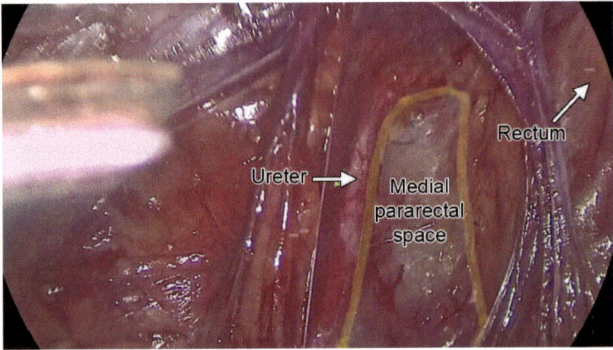

Fig. 7: Left medial pararectal space.

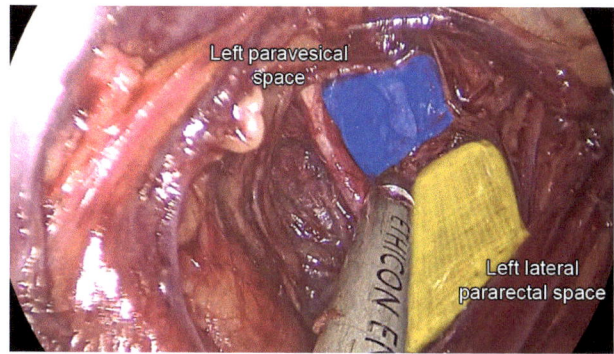

Fig. 8: Left lateral pararectal space.

Yabuki Space

Yoshihiko Yabuki in 2000 was the first described the Yakubi space or the fourth space. It is situated between the cranial portion of the vesicouterine and the ureter.

The space is developed in nerve sparing surgeries as it contains pelvic splanchnic nerves innervating the bladder.

Space of Retzius

Retzius space also called as prevesical or the retropubic space is a small retroperitoneal space situated in the midline between the bladder and the anterior abdominal wall.

It is bounded by:
- Ventrally—pubic symphysis
- Posteriorly—bladder
- Laterally—lateral umbilical ligament

The Retzius space continues laterally into the paravesical spaces on both sides. This space is very useful in surgeries for stress urinary incontinence (SUI) like Burch colposuspension, retropubic tension-free vaginal tapes (TVT), etc. In oncogynecology, this space is entered for anterior exenteration and pelvic anterior peritonectomy. It also forms an important space in surgery for bladder endometriosis.

Vesicovaginal Space/Uterovesical Space

This is a midline space situated between the vagina/cervix posteriorly and the bladder anteriorly. The lateral margins of the space are the vesicouterine ligaments.

In laparoscopic surgery, this space is entered by incising and dissecting the uterovesical peritoneum. These spaces are developed in all cases of hysterectomy and management of deep endometriosis. During dissection, one must always remain above the pubocervical fascia in order to avoid bleeding and stay in the right plane. The dictum that is usually followed is "fat belongs to the bladder".

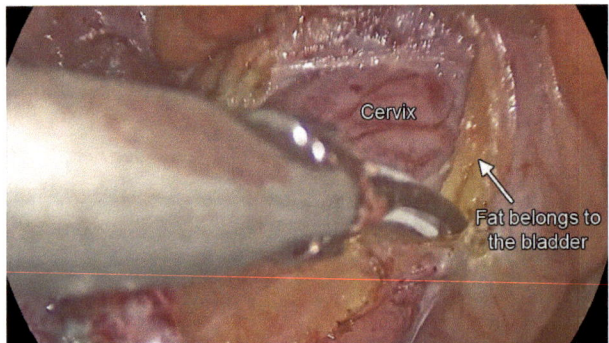

Fig. 9: Vesicovaginal space.

Rectovaginal Space

Rectovaginal space also called the posterior cul de sac is bounded:
- Anteriorly—posterior vaginal wall
- Posteriorly—anterior rectal wall
- Laterally—uterosacral ligaments (cranial) and rectovaginal ligaments (caudal).

This space is exposed in surgeries such as laparoscopic sacrocolpopexy and uterosacral ligament suspension in cases of vaginal vault prolapse, in deep endometriosis, rectovaginal fistula repair, and radical hysterectomy. Injury to the medial rectal artery or the vein and presacral veins can occur if rules of dissection is not followed. The dictum followed here is "fat belongs to the rectum".

Retrorectal Space

Retrorectal space is also called the presacral space. This space is bounded by:
- Anteriorly—rectum
- Posteriorly—sacral promontory, anterior aspect of sacrum, and longitudinal anterior vertebral ligament.
- Laterally—common iliac arteries and ureters

There are three fascial layers of the presacral space—presacral fascia, proper rectal fascia (mesorectal fascia) and Waldeyers fascia. The Waldeyers fascia divides the presacral space into inferior and superior retrorectal space. Identifying these fascial layers are important for different approaches.

In ovarian tumors infiltrating the rectal wall, the interfascial approach between the mesorectal fascia and the presacral area is called the holy plane of dissection. It is useful for total mesorectal excision. Laparoscopic surgeries of endometriosis and for sacrocolpopexy, the transmesorectal approach are used as it avoids serious complications.

CONCLUSION

A sound knowledge of the pelvic anatomy is one of the important aspects for performing safe laparoscopic surgery especially in cases of grade IV endometriosis and pelvic tumors.

Laparoscopy provides an excellent view but with a limited field of vision hence the surgeons need to have a great understanding of the pelvic and its surrounding vicinity.

SUGGESTED READING

1. Alkatout I, Wedel T, Pape J, Possover M, Dhanawat J. Review: Pelvic nerves – from anatomy and physiology to clinical applications. Transl Neurosci. 2021; 12(1):362–78.
2. Ceccaroni M, Pontrelli G, Spagnolo E, et al. Parametrial dissection during laparoscopic nerve-sparing radical hysterectomy: a new approach aims to improve patients' postoperative quality of life. Am J Obstet Gynecol. 2010;202:e1–e2.
3. Fujii S. Anatomic identification of nerve-sparing radical hysterectomy: a step-by-step procedure. Gynecol Oncol. 2008;111:S33–S41.
4. Kostov S, Slavchev S, Dzhenkov D, Mitev D, Yordanov A. Avascular spaces of the female pelvis—clinical applications in obstetrics and gynecology. J Clin Med. 2020;13;9(5):1460.
5. Mirilas P, Skandalakis J. Surgical anatomy of the retroperitoneal spaces part II: the architecture of the retroperitoneal space. Ann Surg. 2010;76:33–42.
6. Yabuki Y, Sasaki H, Hatakeyama N, Murakami G. Discrepancies between classic anatomy and modern gynecologic surgery on pelvic connective tissue structure: harmonization of those concepts by collaborative cadaver dissection. Am J Obstet Gynecol. 2005;193:7–15.
7. Yavuzcan A, Bakay K. Prophylactic ligation of uterine arteries at its origin in laparoscopic surgical staging for endometrial cancer. J Obstet Gynaecol Res. 2021;47(12):4381–88.

CHAPTER 6

Diagnostic Hysteroscopy

Anshu Baser, Archana Baser

Hysteroscopy is perhaps the simplest yet the most hazardous procedure a gynecologist must perform. The most important prerequisites for starting hysteroscopy are—knowledge of uterine and cervical anatomy, instruments, fluid media, managing complications and signs of fluid overload.

PATIENT SELECTION

Hysteroscopy can be offered to the following patients:
- Heavy menstrual bleeding not responding the medical management.
- Suspicious findings on transvaginal sonography (TVS) suggestive of endometrial hyperplasia.
- Failed pipelle biopsy
- Prior to in vitro fertilization
- History of recurrent miscarriages
- Suspected Asherman's syndrome/intrauterine adhesion
- Evaluation of intrauterine fibroids, polyps and septae
- Forgotten missing intrauterine contraceptive device (IUCD).

PATIENT PREPARATION

- Diagnostic hysteroscopy is typically a day procedure. Patients are usually admitted on the morning of the procedure.
- Routine blood investigations and a light meal with an antacid a day before are usually recommended.
- *Antibiotic prophylaxis*: Current recommendations do no support routine antibiotic prophylaxis prior to operative hysteroscopy.[1]
- The most important part omitted in most manuals is the counseling. Diagnostic hysteroscopy although a simple procedure can be disastrous if one does not have sufficient knowledge of uterine anatomy or signs of fluid overload.

Counseling of the patient therefore should include:
- Nature of procedure
- What findings to expect in the procedure
- How will the procedure benefit the patient and its impact on future treatment?

- Possible complications such as perforation or pulmonary edema. This does not mean you scare the patient away. Quote the facts and figures that even though the likelihood of these complications is less yet they are known to occur.
- What will be the postoperative management and care?

PREREQUISITES
- High definition medical grade camera
- High definition endocamera
- Light source (Xenon/LED) and cable
- Recording device.

KNOW YOUR MEDIA

There are various distension media **(Table 1)** available the most popular ones however are normal saline and glycine. With the advent of modern day energy devices normal saline can also be used for distension in diagnostic procedures and switched to operative by using bipolar hysteroscopic devices. It is a common misconception that normal saline is safer than glycine as the rate of absorption in the system under pressure is same for both and therefore fluid balance is of utmost importance. It is important to monitor inflow and outflow.

At regular timed intervals, the values should be reported, and extra vigilance should be paid if there is a discrepancy of more than 500 mL in a healthy patient.

TABLE 1: Comparison of various distension media.[2]

Medium	Advantage	Disadvantage	Risks
CO_2	Safe, easy to use, rapidly absorbed	Poor visibility in the presence of bleeding	CO_2 pulmonary embolism if flow rate exceeds 100 mL/min
Normal saline	Isotonic	Not suitable for monopolar electrosurgery	Fluid overload
Lactated Ringers	Isotonic	Not suitable for monopolar electrosurgery	Fluid overload
Glycine 1.5%	Electrolyte free	Hypotonic	Hypotonic fluid overload
Sorbitol	Nonconductive	Hypotonic	Hyponatremia
Mannitol 5%	Nonconductive	Hypotonic	Hyponatremia
Dextran 32% (Hyskon)	Electrolyte free, nonconductive, immiscible with blood	Highly viscous, difficult to deliver	Hypertonic fluid overload anaphylactic reaction

KNOW YOUR INSTRUMENTS

Many types of hysteroscopes are now available in many sizes. Rigid, semi rigid and flexible scopes are now available.

Flexible Hysteroscopes

These were used in gastrointestinal surgery. They have a deflection control on the body of the scope. The tip can bend up to 120-160 degrees to allow better visualization. Light and image bundles within the scope transmit light into the uterus and return to the eyepiece or video chip. Diagnostic scopes have single channel for the distention medium, while operative hysteroscopes have another channel for instruments. The outer diameter size varies from 3.1 to 5 mm. Narrow diameter and flexible tip enable introduction into the uterine cavity often without anesthesia, which makes it an attractive option.

Rigid Hysteroscopes

Rigid hysteroscopes contain a complex optical telescope element. Glass lenses and spacers are aligned precisely in between the ocular lens (eyepiece) and objective lens at the distal tip. The diameter of the telescope ranges from 1.9 mm (micro hysteroscope) to 4 mm. Viewing angles usually range from 0 to 30 degrees. The outer diameter of the sheath ranges from 3 to 8 mm. Most hysteroscopic systems contain at least one discrete inflow and outflow channel.

Size of Hysteroscope

For diagnostic procedures especially office procedures smaller sized channels are preferred as this reduces the pain and complications. This also reduces the need of cervical dilation and manipulation.

Distension Device

Distension is created either by pressure cuff or hysteromat. Hysteromat allows the fluid to enter the cavity with a specific pressure to minimize the overload of fluid. It has different settings for hysteroscopy and resectoscopic surgeries.

The settings are mostly employed for diagnostic hysteroscopy **(Table 2)**.

PREOPERATIVE PHARMACOLOGICAL AGENTS

Dilatation is usually not required with smaller sized hysteroscopes however, to minimize pain and discomfort; variations in hysteroscopic equipment, use of local anesthesia and use of pharmacological agents have been advocated. The preoperative use of misoprostol or laminar decreases the risk of uterine perforation.[3]

Diagnostic Hysteroscopy

TABLE 2: Routinely employed settings for office hysteroscopy.[4]

Hysteroscope		
• 30° rod lens optic	2.0 mm	2.9 mm
• Diagnostic single-flow sheath	2.8 mm	3.7 mm
• Operative single-flow sheath	3.6 mm	4.3 mm
• Operative continuous-flow sheath	4.2 mm	5.0 mm
Additional instruments and maneuvers		
• Vaginal speculum	Not required	
• Tenaculum	Not required	
• Cervical dilatation	Not required	
Distention medium	Low-viscosity fluids (e.g., saline) with pressure cuff between 80 and 120 mm Hg	
Analgesia/anesthesia	Not required	

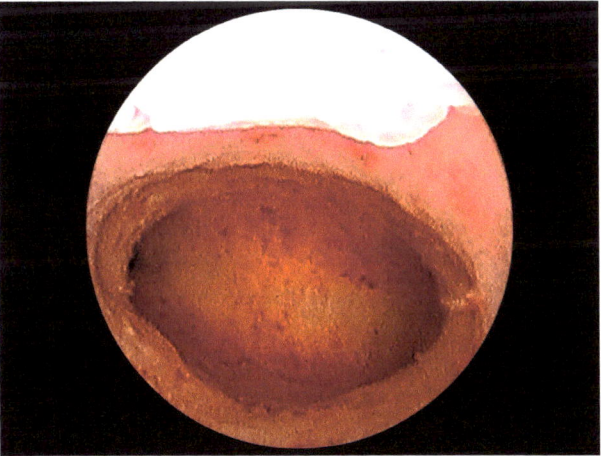

Fig. 1: Normal positioning of ostia with relation to uterine cavity.

PROCEDURE

Hysteroscopy involves introduction of a rigid or flexible hysteroscope via cervix into uterus. It is attached to a camera along with a channel allows the distending media to enter in uterine cavity. Uterine cavity is visualized by contact hysteroscopy. Initially both ostia are inspected, their relation with uterine cavity is also noted. Falloscopy can also be done by flexible hysteroscope **(Fig. 1)**.

■ FINDINGS ON DIAGNOSTIC HYSTEROSCOPY

Müllerian anomalies can lead to abnormal positioning of the ostia. Cornual polyps **(Fig. 2)** are frequently encountered in subfertility patients.

Many submucosal fibroids **(Fig. 3)**, endometrial polyps **(Fig. 4)**, intrauterine adhesions can be very well diagnosed or confirmed in patients with abnormal uterine bleeding **(Fig. 5)**.

Misplaced IUCD is best located by hysteroscopy, also missed fetal bone of second trimester abortion are sometimes picked up **(Fig. 6)**.

Falloposcopy can also be done by flexible hysteroscope. Endometrial tuberculosis can be suspected when caseation seen in cavity **(Fig. 7)** or

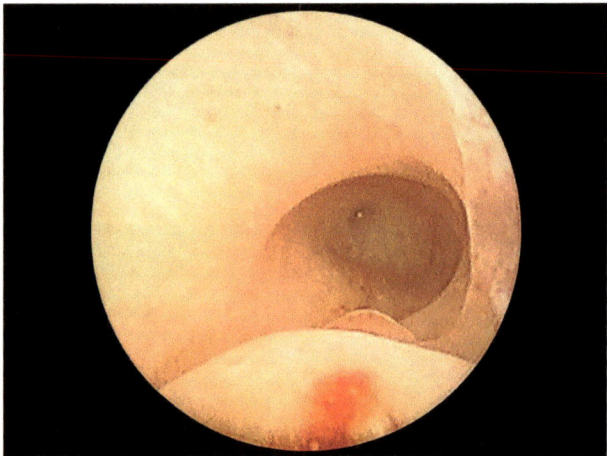

Fig. 2: Unicornuate uterus showing one ostia only.

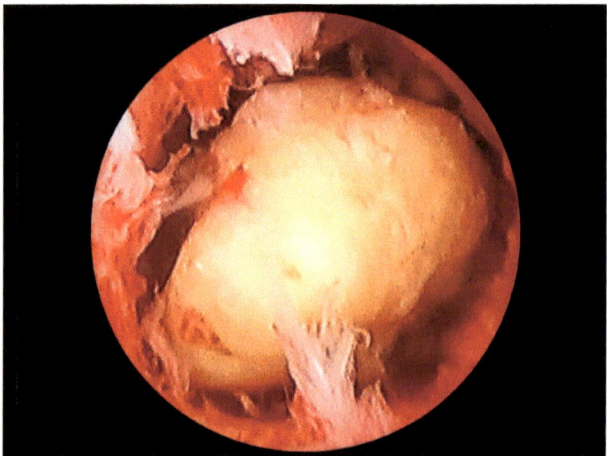

Fig. 3: Submucosal intracavitary fibroid occupying the uterine cavity.

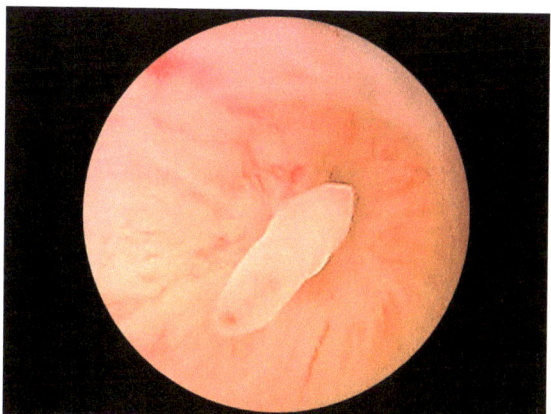
Fig. 4: Cornual polyp obstructing visualization of ostia.

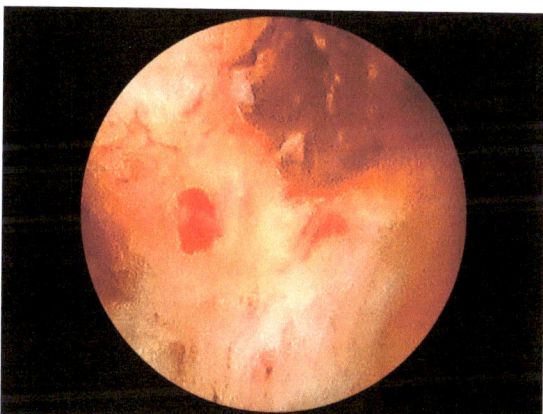
Fig. 5: Dense intrauterine adhesions.

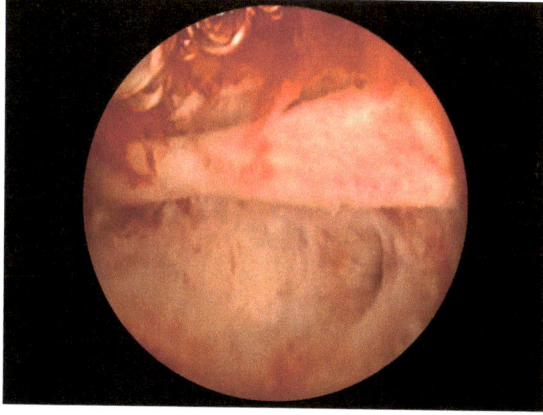
Fig. 6: Missing fetal bone on hysteroscopy.

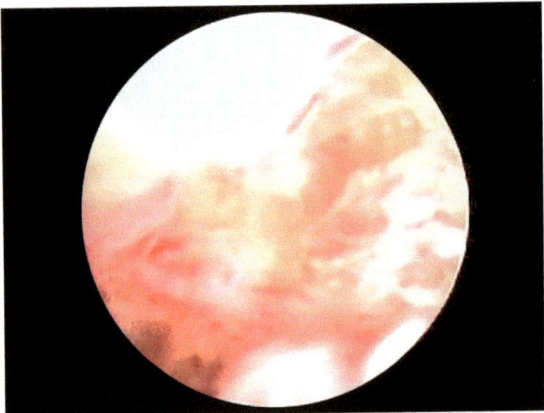

Fig. 7: Caseation noted in cavity along with irregular endometrial cavity in a case of endometrial TB.

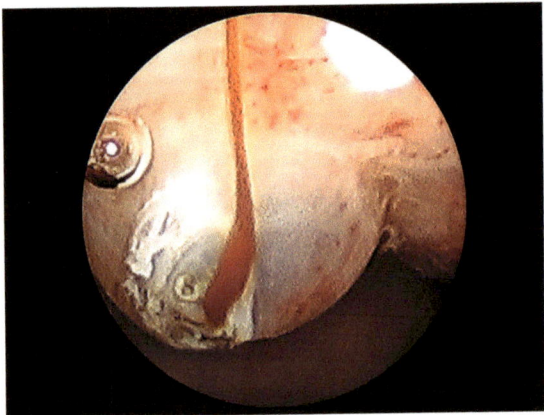

Fig. 8: Endometriotic cyst with chocolate fluid coming out.

tubercles are noted. Endometritis is another common finding. A rare endometriotic cyst with chocolate fluid coming can be best picked by hysteroscopy **(Fig. 8)**.

■ OFFICE HYSTEROSCOPY

Outpatient hysteroscopy, whether diagnostic or operative is successful, safe and well tolerated. However, as with any procedure requiring instrumentation of the uterus, outpatient hysteroscopy can be associated with significant pain and anxiety. Expert preoperative evaluation is essential in determining the surgical skill and expertise needed, surgical time, and the likelihood of completing the operative procedure. Overall, complications in outpatient hysteroscopy are infrequent. Sometimes, the office hysteroscopy procedure is failed due to cervical stenosis, pain and poor visualization.

COMPLICATIONS OF HYSTEROSCOPY

Complications of both diagnostic and operative hysteroscopy are rare, however they do occur. Common complications are:
- Uterine perforation (0.12%)
- Fluid overload (0.06%)
- Intraoperative hemorrhage (0.03%)
- Bladder or bowel injury (0.02%)
- Endomyometritis (0.01%)

KEY MESSAGE

There is now increase in uptake and awareness regarding hysteroscopy amongst gynecologists. Our continuous enthusiasm has led to advancements in techniques as well as instrumentation.

Basic knowledge of procedure, instruments and potential complications can avoid mishaps in this procedure and improve future outcomes.

REFERENCES

1. Muzii L, Di Donato V, Boni T, Gaglione R, Marana R, Mazzon I, et al. Antibiotics prophylaxis for operative hysteroscopy. Reprod Sci. 2017;24(4):534-38.
2. Bieber EJ, Sanfilippo JS, Horowitz IR, Shafi MI. Laparoscopic and hysteroscopic instrumentation. Clin Gynecol. 2015; 589-603.
3. Al-Fozan H, Firwana B, Al Kadri H, Hassan S, Tulandi T. Preoperative ripening of the cervix before operative hysteroscopy. Cochrane Database Syst Rev. 2015; 23(4):CD005998.
4. Bettocchi S, Achilarre M, Ceci O, Luigi, S. Fertility-Enhancing Hysteroscopic Surgery. Seminars in Reproductive Medicine. 2011;29(2):75-082.

CHAPTER 7

Complications in Laparoscopy

B Ramesh, Jasmine S Abraham

Complications can occur in any surgery, but it is necessary to anticipate and take appropriate measure to resolve it. Also knowledge on how to prevent complication is very important.

- *Anesthesia-related complications:*
  - Prolonged ventilation for difficult incubation especially in women with short neck on obesity—leads to stomach distention—therefore it is important to use RT to deflate stomach before verses or trocar use.
  - Patients are prone to hypoxia, alveolar atelectasis due to steep Trendelenburg position.
  - Also reduces venous return prone to deep vein thrombosis (DVT).
  - Extraperitoneal gas insufflation.
  - Subcutaneous emphysema 0.3–3%.
  - Needs in subcutaneous plane or in prolonged procedures.
  - Resolve in 12–24 hours.
- *Patient position-related complications:*
  - More in slender patient, diabetes.
  - Common peroneal nerve injury, femoral nerve, brachial nerve plexus injury.
  - Prevention:
    - Common peroneal nerve—use both stirrups.
    - Common femoral nerve—maintain hip flexes 60–110°, knee flexion 90–120°, hip abduction <90° manual hip rotation.
    - Brachial flexes injury—one arm can be tricked closed to patient and other <90° abduction.
- *Air embolism:*
  - Rare.
  - Intravascular entry of gas.
  - Air embolism can cause gas block in inferior vena cava (IVC) and right atrium-reduced cardiac output-arrest.
  - Can also cause increased right ventricle hypertension and paradoxical gas embolism.

- Signs are tachycardia, arrhythmia hypotension, more cerebral vein thrombosis (CVT), murmurs—mill wheel murmur, cyanosis, right heart strain on ECG, hypoxia.
- Can be associate with pulmonary edema.
- $PETCO_2$ due to below cardiac output.
- Aspiration of gas/foamy blood in central line establishes diagnosis.

TREATMENT

- Immediate stop insufflation.
- Straighten OT table and move to head low and left lateral decubitus position.
- Ventilate with 100% moist oxygen.
- May use central venous catheter to aspirate gas.
- External Cardiac massage may help in fragmenting CO_2 bubbles.
    - *Electrosurgical injuries:*
        - *Insulation failure:* Always check insulation before every surgery to prevent this.
        - *Direct coupling:* When an active instrument comes in contact with another instrument.
        - Prevent this by activating under vision.
        - *Capacitation coupling:* In monopolar mode on alternate current may induce a counter through the insulation to an instrumental in close proximity.
        - Can eliminate this problem with use of bipolar.
        - *Dispersive electrode pad:* Misapplication of the pad can result in thermal burns.
        - Whole surface area of pad must be in contact with skin and pad must be placed closed to operating site.
        - Avoid placing over bony prominences, dense fat (buttocks) ++hairy skin.
        - Upper thigh is an ideal site for abdominal surgery.
        - Vascular injury:
            - Abdominal wall vessel
            - Large retroperitoneal vessel

Abdominal wall vessel injury: Most common inferior epigastric vessel 3/1000 operative laparoscopy is the incidence.

Inferior epigastric artery injury:
- Bipolar coagulation
- Tamponade—No. 14 Foley's catheter
- Suturing.

Prevention of inferior epigastric injury:
- Insert trocar in lower quadrant lateral to rectus muscle.
- Careful inspection of peritoneum of anterior abdomen wall.

Large retroperitoneal vessel injury: Include aorta, vena cava, iliac vessels.
- May be sustained during insertion of verses or primary trocar.

Presentation—sudden drop in BP:
- Gush of blood from verse/trocar.
- Hemorrhage seen following laparoscope.

MANAGEMENT

Veress/trocar must not be removed as it will act as plug to prevent massive blood, also helps to identify site of injury.
- Immediate resuscitation with simultaneous laparotomy must be done.
- Apply pressure over defect/unable to identify pressure over aorta.
- Seek assistance from vascular surgeon.

PREVENTION OF VASCULAR INJURY

Adhere to safe laparoscopic entry technique.
- Have a routine practice to palpate abdomen before port placement.
- Trocar must be sharp.
- Gentle, controlled entry.
- Direction of Veress and primary trocar must be toward hollow of sacrum and not sidewards.
- All secondary ports placed under vision.

Bowel injury: 55% occurred during abdominal access.

Cause: Laceration.

Thermal injury: Direct burn/coupling—direct and capacitator

Recognition of tip of Veress/trocar has entered bowel lumen, foul smelling greenish fluid will be seen from open end of needle.

In through and through perspiration—can result if segment adherent to anterior abdominal wall.

Thus may escape detention.

To check—withdraw laparoscope into trocar sleeve and check if injury has occurred—bowel lumen will be seen.

MANAGEMENT

Veress needle prick—expectant.
- *Trocar injury*: Leave tip in lumen, proceed with laboratory.
    - If small bowel is involved—primary closure on layers.
    - If large bowel is injured—(1) Primary repair, (2) Colostomy, (3) Segment resection.

Complications in Laparoscopy

- If thermal injury—resection may be needed.
  - Delayed presentation—4–10 days after thermal injury.
  - Pain abdomen, distention forming fever.
  - Peritonitis features later.

PREVENTION OF BOWEL INJURY

Use safely techniques
- Use RT
- Bowel preparation
- Port site hernia—can present within O_2 seeks with swelling.
  - Can miss diagnose of fascia and rectus.
  - *Prevention:* Probe >7 mm—closure of fascia and rectus hematoma.
- Port site metastasis
  - *Prevention:* Endology/wound protector.

CHAPTER 8

Complications in Hysteroscopy

S Krishnakumar, Aditi Abhade

INTRODUCTION

In the past 20-30 years, hysteroscopy has revolutionized the treatment of benign uterine disorders and the procedure has found wide acceptance among gynecologists in their routine practice. As the usage of hysteroscopy for diagnostic and operative purposes has risen, it is of utmost importance to be aware of the associated complications and the measures for their management. Though the complication rates of hysteroscopy are low, varying from 0.013% for diagnostic hysteroscopy to 0.28% for operative procedures, the art of hysteroscopy requires training and experience. Moreover, safety and outcome of surgical procedures are clearly linked to adequate training and adherence to safety recommendations. Also, the adoption of possible preventive measures will help in increasing the quality and safety of hysteroscopic surgeries.

CLASSIFICATION

The complications associated with hysteroscopy can be broadly divided into intraoperative and postoperative complications or into those related with purely diagnostic procedures and those related to operative procedures. A recently proposed system groups the complications into specific 'Adverse event categories' **(Table 1)**.

We will restrict to the following complications, specific to hysteroscopic surgery for want of space.

MEDIA AND DISTENSION-RELATED COMPLICATIONS

Uterine cavity requires distension to visualize and perform surgeries and today for all practical reasons only liquid distension media are used and we shall restrict to the use of low-viscosity media in the modern hysteroscopy of which the most common are the Glycine, normal saline and Ringers lactate. Moreover, with the shift of hysteroscopy to the office setting, use of miniature sheaths, possibility of performing almost 80% of procedures with bipolar energy devices, the latter two types of fluid media have replaced the use of Glycine 1.5% in modern practice. With available evidence on safety, one can now propagate the use of the electrolyte containing, iso-osmotic saline and ringers lactate for all hysteroscopic procedures.

TABLE 1: Adverse event categories.

Patient positioning	Neurological compartment syndrome
Anesthesia	• General • Regional • Conscious sedation • Local
Access to the uterine cavity	• Cervical trauma • Perforations
Distension medium	• Gas embolism • Fluid overload • Electrolyte imbalances
Perforations	• Uterus • Adjacent structures (bowel, bladder, vessels)
Bleeding	• Cervical • Endometrial • From pelvic vessels
Electrosurgery	• Local (active electrodes) • Distant (current diversion)
Infections	• Endomyometritis • Peritonitis
Late complications	• Intrauterine adhesions (synechiae) • Obstetric complications (uterine rupture, placenta accreta/increta, etc.).

TABLE 2: Electrolyte content and osmolality.

Solution	Na mEq/L	Cl mEq/L	mOsm/L
0.9% Sodium chloride	154	154	308
Lactated Ringer's	130	110	275
0.45% Sodium chloride	77	77	155
3% Sorbitol	–	–	178
1.5% Glycine	–	–	200
5% Mannitol	–	–	275
5% Dextrose in water	–	–	250

The categories, features and safety profile of various types of distending media are shown in **Table 2**.

1.5% glycine was the commonest medium used in conventional hysteroscopic surgical procedures involving resectoscopic electrosurgery. With the introduction of smaller operative sheaths, majority of the procedures can be done without the resectoscope. This, combined with the availability of good bipolar energy devices has considerably reduced the need for glycine in hysteroscopic procedures. Glycine is a nonconductive amino acid with a plasma half-life of 85 minutes and is hypo-osmolar. It is uniquely metabolized in the liver to ammonia and free water, which can result in further reduction of serum osmolality. Ammonia may add to the consequences of excess absorption, as in such instances, coma has been described despite the correction of electrolyte disturbances.

Normal saline (NS) and other isotonic electrolyte-rich solutions are useful and safe media, for even if there is substantial systemic absorption, they do not cause electrolyte imbalance and consequently are a good choice for minor procedures performed in the office. While electrolyte-containing solutions are not suitable for RF surgery with monopolar RF systems, the development of bipolar RF instrumentation for hysteroscopic surgery has allowed the application of saline as a distending medium in even more advanced and complex procedures. Ringer's lactate, while infrequently reported as a medium used for hysteroscopy, possesses similar properties as normal saline but is even more "physiologic" and consequently would be expected to have a similar risk profile. However, no studies were identified that specifically evaluated the use of Ringer's lactate for hysteroscopy. It should be borne in mind that isotonic saline or Ringer's lactate, if absorbed in sufficient volume, has been associated with fluid overload leading to right-sided heart failure and pulmonary edema.

Excess absorption of distension media is one of the most frequent complications in operative hysteroscopy. Especially when using monopolar electrosurgical instruments, electrolyte-containing fluid is incompatible, and where 1.5% glycine is used, it can lead to dilutional hyponatremia and hypo-osmalilty. These conditions may have catastrophic consequences if they are not recognized promptly. The brain swells as it attempts to become isosmotic with the vascular system. If swelling exceeds 5%, the risk of severe neurological damage dramatically increases. This problem gets exaggerated in premenopausal women because of the inhibition of the sodium pump. Classic clinical features of hyponatremic hypovolemia include apprehension, confusion, fatigue, headache, mental agitation, nausea, visual disturbances, vomiting and weakness. These complications are more readily apparent when regional anesthesia is used rather than general anesthesia.

GUIDELINES FOR DISTENSION MEDIA

1. Use bipolar resectoscope, where isotonic, electrolytic fluid, Ringer's lactate or 0.9% saline can be used.
2. Draw preoperative serum electrolytes for a baseline in all patients, undergoing major monopolar resectoscopic surgery and evaluate electrolytes (Na), status of procedure, patients condition, if deficit >1,000 mL.
3. Continuously record inflow and outflow using the electronic monitor with deficit alarm set at 750 mL.

4. Discuss with the anesthetist (e.g., procedure, IV fluids, vital signs, pulse oximetry, patient's risks).
5. Consider epidural anesthesia in high-risks patients.
6. Stop procedure if deficit is >1,500 mL, electrolytes decrease, and there are signs of decompression.

The best distension devices for hysteroscopic procedures are the automated pumps as shown in **Figure 1**, but if these are not available one can use 2 Medex bags with TUR set for continuous flow of media **(Fig. 2)**.

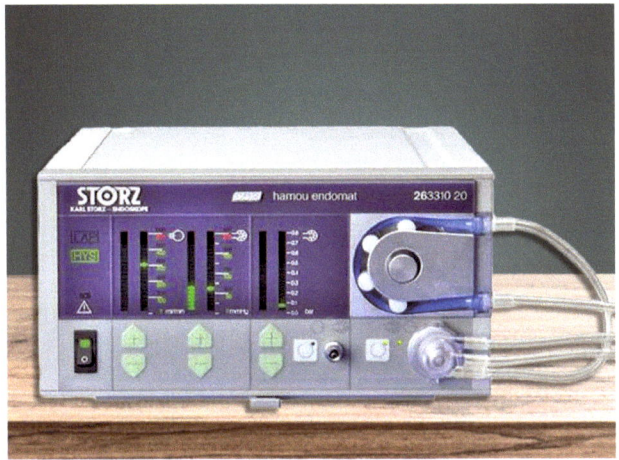

Fig. 1: Automated pump.

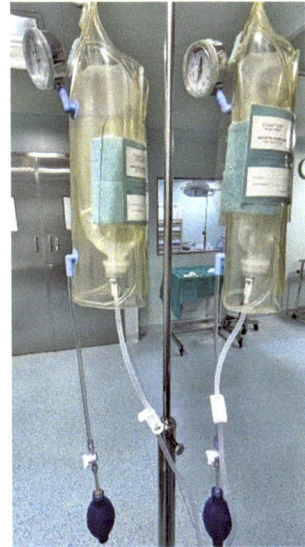

Fig. 2: Medex bags with transurethra resection (TUR) set for continuous flow of media.

If electronic device is not present in the operation theater, one attendant should be given the job of monitoring the amount of liquid infused and the amount that is drained in the suction bottle, and he should warn the surgeon of the deficit. Keep the distension fluid at body temperature and monitor the patient's core temperature continuously. If the fluid deficit reaches 750 mL, immediately give 20-40 mg of intravenous frusemide and draw a sample for serum electrolytes. Interrupt the procedure for 5-10 minutes to allow the uterus to contact and to seal off small blood vessels. Discontinue the procedure if the fluid deficit reaches 1,500 mL or if the serum sodium level is below 125 mEq/L. The use of bipolar devices in normal saline prevents dilutional hyponatremia, but fluid deficits must still be monitored. Large fluid deficits can lead to pulmonary edema and death.

GAS EMBOLISM

Sources of gas embolism are room air, carbon dioxide, carbon monoxide, and other gaseous products of combustion. The anesthetist will be the first person to identify the following signs:
- Sudden fall in oxygen saturation
- Sudden hypotension
- Hypercarbia
- Arrhythmias
- Tachypnea or a mill wheel murmur

If gas embolism develops, immediately stop the procedure and ventilate the patient with 100% oxygen. To reduce risk of gas embolism:
- Avoid Trendelenburg positioning.
- Remove last dilator just before inserting the resectoscope.
- Limit repeated removal-reinsertion of the resectoscope.
- Vaporizing myomas eliminates the need to remove fibroids.
- Intracervical injection of vasopressin may block gas from entering the circulation.

TRAUMATIC LESIONS AND THEIR PREVENTION

Traumatic lesions are more common with hysteroscopic procedures carried out in an operating room, but may also be seen in the ambulatory setting. These comprise of uterine perforation, injury to bowel or bladder and the creation of false passages. Predisposing factors of traumatic lesions are:
- Cervical stenosis as seen in nulliparous patients, postmenopausal age group and history of previous surgeries on the cervix.
- Uterine anomalies.
- Severe uterine anteflexion or retroflexion
- Uterine hypoplasia
- Endometrial carcinoma.

Traumatic injuries may occur due to cervical dilatation, the hysteroscope, or due to instruments or electrosurgical devices. Entry injuries can be totally avoided by learning to insert the hysteroscope under vision with the smaller Bettocchi sheaths of 4 mm or 5 mm with either 2 mm or 2.9 mm telescopes respectively. The smaller diameter sheaths now commonly used is shown in **Figures 3 and 4**.

One must learn to follow the hysteroscopic anatomy from external os to the cervical mucosal folds which all converge to the internal os and can be labeled as the GEM point (getting entry methodically). Dilatation is blind and the modern available sheaths totally have replaced the need of dilation of cervix unless one has to use the resectoscope. But with the availability of smaller diameter resectoscopes from 15 French has replaced the need for dilatation even in resectoscopic surgeries **(Fig. 5)**.

Most uterine perforations, even those involving large dilators, usually do not require treatment, but further assessment may be required to rule out bowel injury. When perforation occurs during the use of thermal energy, laparoscopy is necessary to assess the organs overlying the site. Intraoperative bleeding is more common when endometrial or fibroid resection is

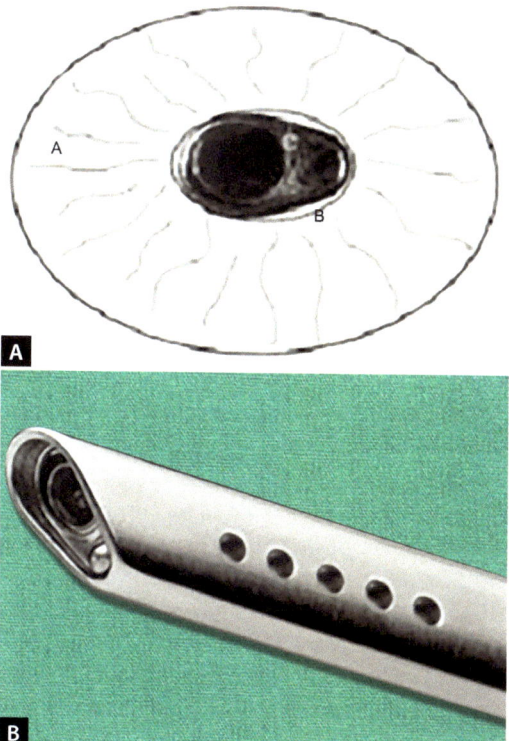

Figs. 3A and B

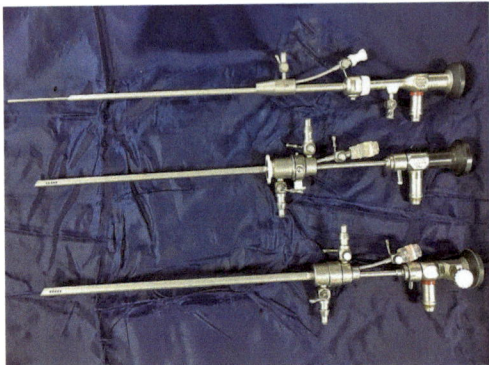

Fig. 4

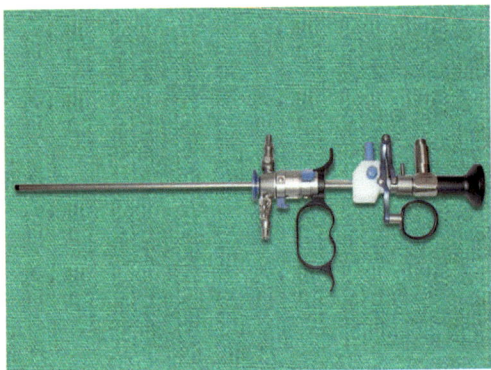

Fig. 5: Resectoscope

performed with loop electrode. Bleeding sufficient to require intervention occurs at a rate of 0.5–1.9% in several reported series. To achieve hemostasis, the vessels can be coagulated if seen. If a bleeder is not identifiable, one can either pack the uterus with ribbon gauze soaked with diluted vasopressin, or a Foley's catheter with balloon inflated with 15–20 mL of fluid is kept for 2 hours. To reduce intraoperative bleeding during operative hysteroscopy, Philips demonstrated a marked decrease in blood loss by injecting very dilute vasopressin (0.2 mL) in 60 mL of normal saline, directly into the cervix 2 cm deep, at the 4 and 8 o'clock positions. A vaporizing electrode may prevent significant blood loss during myoma resection (Versapoint). Preoperative danazol or GnRH agonists decrease the thickness and vascularity of the endometrium and shrink fibroids.

Perforation with an active electrode occurs when current is applied as the electrode is extended or the resectoscope is moved toward the fundus. It can be avoided if the electrode is activated only when moving it toward the operator. Diversion of current occurs when electrode insufflation fails, which allows current to jump to the outer sheath of the resectoscope. To avoid this, inspect all the electrodes thoroughly before surgery. To avoid return-pad injuries, keep the patient's thigh completely dry, ensure that the pad is flat against the skin at application. A major step towards safety will be to switch to using bipolar resectoscopes and a generator which generates bipolar cutting current.

GENERAL ASPECTS FOR SAFETY DURING HYSTEROSCOPY

- *Initial evaluation*: Every patient requires a complete preoperative evaluation starting with thorough history and physical examination. All appropriate laboratory investigations should be carried out and a good transvaginal sonography should be carried out before complex surgical procedures. If indicated hysterograms can be carried out and viewed by the surgeon.
- *Concurrent laparoscopy*: Simultaneous laparoscopy is indicated in:
  - Infertility evaluation
  - Congenital anomalies of uterus
  - Tubal cannulation for blocked fallopian tube
- *Preparation of endometrium*: Plan all surgeries within the uterine cavity in the early proliferative phase of the cycle. In patients with endometrial hyperplasia, waiting for transcervical resection of endometrium (TCRE), the endometrium can be prepared by gonadotropin-releasing hormone or oral contraceptive (OC) pills.
- Learn to do simple operative procedures first after being comfortable with hysteroscopic anatomy and diagnostic procedure. The simplest procedure to perform will be small septum, small polyps and the moving on to larger septum, submucous myomas and lastly intrauterine adhesions.
- *Video hysteroscopy*: Needless to say all operative procedures should be done with a good camera system and complete recording of the procedure.

For prolonged procedures, it is advisable to dedicate an operation theater attendant to accurately record and read out the quantity of liquid medium used and the volume recovered. Additionally it is important to inform the anesthesiologist about side effects of selected medium prior to surgery. It is always advisable to use isotonic electrolyte containing liquid media (Ringer's lactate, 0.9% saline) for distension. Bipolar current if available should be the current of choice whenever electrosurgery is planned.

DO'S AND DON'TS IN HYSTEROSCOPIC SURGERY

Do's

- Always select the patients properly, paying attention to indications and contraindications.
- Counsel the patient properly, regarding the procedure being attempted, their realistic results, and the associated complications.

- Get all the investigations necessary, like hysterosalpingography (HSG), transvaginal sonography and have them evaluated just prior to the beginning of the surgery.
- Keep all the equipment and instruments ready, before the surgery. The surgeon must know to assemble and dismantle all the instruments himself and check their smooth functioning, just before the commencement of the surgery. Use standard instruments and equipment.
- Follow all the safety precautions recommended, like the inflow pressure, current settings, etc.
- Use isotonic electrolyte containing solutions for all hysteroscopic surgeries.
- Switch over to bipolar current as modality of choice in resectoscopic surgeries. If using monopolar current, always use non-ionic electrolyte free solutions.
- Have an attendant dedicated for monitoring the fluid deficit in all hysteroscopic surgeries.
- Avoid, Trendelenburg position during hysteroscopic surgeries.
- Use cervical softening agents like vaginal misoprostol for easy cervical dilatation
- Before embarking upon difficult surgeries like intrauterine adhesiolysis, submucous myoma resection, do sufficient diagnostic and simple hysteroscopic surgeries, to be well adjusted to all the steps.
- At the beginning of the surgery, always inspect the cavity of the uterus and identify the normal uterine anatomy.
- In the event of fluid overload, other complications abandon the procedure, identify the complication and immediately rectify them.
- Always remember the surgery can be completed at a second sitting.
- Keep proper record of all the procedure done and document all steps.
- Inform the patient about all the complications if any and the need for subsequent follow-up.

Don'ts

- Do not start surgery if instruments are malfunctioning.
- Do not use unsafe pressure devices for delivering fluid.
- Do not give deep head low positions.
- Do not over dilate the cervix.
- Do not begin or continue surgery if the anatomy is not clear.
- Do not use electrolyte containing solutions for monopolar resectoscopic surgeries.
- Do not exceed the recommended fluid the deficit during hysteroscopic surgeries.

CHAPTER 9
Sterilization and Disinfection in Endoscopy

Subash Mallya

INTRODUCTION

Laparoscopic surgeries are becoming more and more common since more than two decades. A major risk of all such procedures is the introduction of pathogens that can lead to infection. Failure to properly disinfect or sterilize equipment carries risk for person-to-person transmission (e.g., hepatitis B virus) and transmission of environmental pathogens (e.g., *Pseudomonas aeruginosa*).

The laparoscopic instruments are more complex in design and yet delicate in construction. Thus, the laparoscopic instruments are more vulnerable to lodging of bioburden (microorganisms and debris) within their crevices. Laparoscopic instruments are difficult to clean, sterilize adequately and maintain as compared to their counterparts used in open surgery.

Factors that Affect the Efficacy of both Disinfection and Sterilization

- Prior cleaning of the object l organic and inorganic load present
- Type and level of microbial contamination
- Concentration of and exposure time to the germicide
- Physical nature of the object (e.g., crevices, hinges, and lumens)
- Temperature and pH of the disinfection process

CLEANING, DISINFECTING, AND STERILIZING OF ENDOSCOPIC INSTRUMENTS

The initial and most important step of reprocessing is thorough cleaning to remove gross soil, including microorganisms (bioburden), which allows the disinfectant or sterilizing agents to work effectively. Organic materials may inactivate these agents or present a barrier that prevents disinfectants from reaching all surfaces of an instrument. Manual cleaning is the safest method to use for rigid and single-lumen flexible endoscopes and accessories. Ultrasonic washers can damage and loosen small joints and remove adhesives and lubricants. Enzymatic detergents are excellent choices for cleaning endoscopic instruments. The enzymes used in these detergents are specific to protein, sugar, or fat.

Sterilization

Steam is the most common and least expensive method of sterilization. However, many lensed endoscopic instruments cannot be steam sterilized. Even instruments and telescopes marketed as "autoclavable" will last longer if processed by alternative methods. Heat-sensitive objects can be treated with ethylene oxide (EtO), hydrogen peroxide gas plasma; or if other methods are unsuitable, by liquid *chemical sterilants*.

EtO Sterilization

Ethylene oxide gas has been the standard for sterilizing heat-sensitive items, including endoscopes. Sterilization cycles are typically one and one-half to 2 hours at 55°C. Items must then be aerated mechanically for 8 to 12 hours. EtO is being gradually replaced in some hospitals with other sterilization methods, such as steam, vapor-phase methods, and per acetic acid because of cost and safety concerns. The Steris system (Steris, Mentor, Ohio) uses per acetic acid in a proprietary liquid processor to sterilize items in less than 30 minutes at 50–55°C. This method is a just-in-time process and sterility cannot be maintained for long-term storage. Plasma and/or vapor phase are another sterilization modality for endoscopic instruments. STERRAD (Advanced Sterilization Processes of Irvine, Calif.) is FDA-approved for use in the US.

Disinfection

If sterilization is not possible, high-level disinfection is recommended for laparoscopes and hand instruments that come in contact with peritoneum and the live tissue. High-level disinfectants are sporicidal, bactericidal, virucidal, and fungicidal agents that remove most bioburden, with the exception of some spores.

Germicides categorized as chemical sterilants:
- Glutaraldehyde (>2.4%)-based formulations
- Glutaraldehyde (0. 95%) with phenol/phenate (1.64%)
- Stabilized hydrogen peroxide (7.5%)
- Hydrogen peroxide (7.35%) with peracetic acid (0.23%)
- Peracetic acid (0.2%)
- Peracetic acid (0.08%) with hydrogen peroxide (1.0%)

Commercial preparations of glutaraldehyde are available in both alkaline and acidic formulations. Although the slightly acidic preparations appear to be safe for endoscopic instrumentation, alkaline preparations are more common. The solutions are available in 2.4% or 3.5% concentrations. The 2.4% concentrations without surfactants are the recommended solutions for endoscopic instruments.

After the instruments having been disinfected they require rinsing with sterile water. Rinsing endoscopes and flushing channels with sterile water, filtered water, or tap water will prevent adverse effects associated with disinfectant retained in the endoscope (e.g., disinfectant-induced peritonitis). Glutaraldehyde manufacturers are now recommending three separate, sterile rinses of at least 1 minute each. The rinse water is not to be reused.

ISSUES CONTRIBUTING TO IMPROPER CLEANING

In any facility, the challenges include:
- Keeping instruments free of gross soil during the surgical procedure
- Minimizing the length of time between instruments leaving the surgical field and the beginning of the cleaning process having the right cleaning equipment and solutions in the right place.

A brief summary of the proper steps would include following points:
- Begin the cleaning process as soon as the procedure is done. Proteins in blood and other tissue can dry and cake on the internal as well as external surfaces of a device; when this happens, thorough cleaning is difficult, if not impossible.
- Covering the instruments with a wet cloth is not enough to keep them from drying out. The best approach is to place the instruments in a basin of solution that is waiting for them when they come off the surgical table.
- Wipe down surfaces of instruments with an enzymatic solution. Flush lumens in laparoscopic instruments and accessories to remove gross debris.
- Separate general surgical instruments from specialized or more delicate instruments.
- Transport instruments to the specified cleaning area. Clean and sterilize according to manufacturers' written instructions.

OPERATION THEATER—DISCIPLINE

- Only people absolutely needed for an assigned work should be present.
- People present in theater should make minimal movements and curtail unnecessary movements in and out of theaters, which will greatly reduce bacterial count.
- Airborne contamination is usually affected by type of surgery, quality of air which in fact depends on rate of air exchange.
- Prompt disposal of theater waste out of the theater is of top priority. Any spillage of body fluids including blood on the floors is highly hazardous and prompts the rapid multiplication of nosocomial pathogens in particular *Pseudomonas* spp.

STERILIZATION AND DISINFECTION OF OPERATION THEATERS AND CRITICAL CARE AREAS

General Instructions

- Keep the floor dry when in use.
- Use only vacuum cleaners (booming to be forbidden as it will dispense the infected material all around and on the equipment.
- Chemical disinfection of an operation room floor is probably unnecessary. The bacteria carrying particles already on the floor are unlikely to reach an open wound in sufficient numbers to cause an infection (Ayliffe et al. 1967, Hombroeus et al. 1978). Cleaning alone followed by drying will considerably reduce bacterial population.
- *Wall and ceilings:* Wall and ceilings are rarely contaminated. The numbers of bacteria do not appear to increase even if walls are not cleaned. Frequent cleaning is not necessary and has little influence on bacterial counts. Routine disinfection is therefore unnecessary, but only cleaned when dirty.

Laparoscopes

Although high-level disinfection appears to be the minimum standard for processing laparoscopes between patients, this practice continues to be debated. Proponents of high-level disinfection refer to membership surveys or institutional experiences involving more than 117,000 and 10,000 laparoscopic procedures, respectively, that cite a low risk for infection when high-level disinfection is used for gynecological laparoscopic instruments.

Disinfection of HBV-, HCV-, HIV- or TB-contaminated Devices

The Centers for Disease Control and Prevention (CDC) recommendation for high-level disinfection of HBV-, HCV-, HIV or TB-contaminated devices is appropriate because experiments have demonstrated the effectiveness of high-level disinfectants to inactivate these and other pathogens that might contaminate semi-critical devices. Endoscopes and other semicritical devices should be managed the same way regardless of whether the patient is known to be infected with HBV, HCV, HIV or *M. tuberculosis*.

An evaluation of a manual disinfection procedure to eliminate HCV from experimentally-contaminated endoscopes provided some evidence that cleaning and 2% glutaraldehyde for 20 minutes should prevent transmission. The inhibitory activity of a phenolic and a chlorine compound on HCV showed that the phenolic inhibited the binding and replication of HCV, but the chlorine was ineffective, probably because of its low concentration and its neutralization in the presence of organic matter.

CONCLUSION

The knowledge on maintenance, sterilization and control of infections in operation theaters is a rapidly evolving science. Reusable endoscopic instruments can be reprocessed safely and effectively, providing they are cleaned and sterilized or disinfected according to the manufacturers' recommendations. All cleaning, disinfecting and sterilizing processes must be standardized and monitored to ensure process quality and specific policies and procedures established to ensure proper handling and standardized practices.

SUGGESTED READING

1. Garner JS, Favero MS. Guidelines for handwashing and hospital environmental control. Am J Infect Control. 1985;14:110-126.
2. Good hospital practice: Handling and biological decontamination of reusable medical devices (American National Standard) designation. Arl ington, VA; Association for the Advancement of Medical Instrumentation; 1992.pp.669-90.
3. Milner NA. A system approach to patient-safe rigid and flexible endoscopes: A microbiologist's point of view. J Healthcare Material Management.1992;10:3. Young EC. A disinfectant guide. Urologic Nursing. 1990. pp.9-7.
4. Reichert M, Patterson P. Endoscopes: Tough problems with their cleaning and reprocessing. OR Manager. 1990;6:1-7.
5. Russel AD, Hugo WB, Ayliffe GAJ. Principles and Practice of Disinfection, Preservation and Sterilization.

CHAPTER 10

Myoma Specimen Retrieval Methods

Pandit Palaskar

Minimally invasive surgical techniques involve small laparoscopic incisions which make tissue extraction a challenge. The problem of specimen removal during minimally invasive procedures led to the development of tissue morcellation techniques. Morcellation refer to any surgical technique involving fragmenting a surgical specimen into smaller pieces that can be removed through small incisions. Myoma morcellation has gained attention in recent years due to the controversy regarding its use in cases of myomas with rare possibility of occult sarcoma.

CATEGORIES OF TISSUE MORCELLATION

Currently there are three general categories of tissue morcellation (AAGL):
1. Vaginal morcellation through a posterior colpotomy
2. Minilaparotomy/laparoendoscopic single site (LESS) morcellation
3. Electromechanical morcellation (EMM)

The former two approaches have been used for decades, but it is not known at this time if they share equivalent risks as EMM regarding dissemination of an occult malignancy. Each technique outlined above can be performed within a specimen retrieval bag.

Extirpation of uterine tissue through the vagina or minilaparotomy, even with the aid of manual morcellation, may limit tissue-scattering effects and has been shown to be safe with outcomes comparable to electromechanical morcellation in avoiding the need for laparotomy.[1]

Vaginal Morcellation

Method: It involves incision over the posterior vaginal wall which can be made more prominent by vaginal obturator or tube. The myoma is pushed through the colpotomy incision laparoscopically and pulled vaginally with help of Allis forceps or Vulsellum. The vagina can accommodate removal of bulky tissue after posterior colpotomy, providing a single, concealed incision. This technique is safe with outcomes comparable or superior to traditional extirpation methods.[2]

A large uterus with a narrow pelvic arch and obese patients makes transvaginal tissue removal challenging, but several maneuvers may be used by skilled gynecologic surgeons to facilitate this process. A vaginal retractor with long instruments can provide appropriate exposure.[3] For large specimens, tissue morcellation techniques including bivalving, coring and wedge resection can be performed within a specimen retrieval bag[4] have been utilized for the past century and newer techniques such as the "paper roll" method have been described.[5]

A randomized trial comparing transumbilical with transvaginal specimen removal after adnexectomy demonstrated less pain in those removed transvaginally with no difference in dyspareunia or infectious or wound complications.[2]

Minilaparotomy or Laparoendoscopic Single Site Morcellation

In today's era of minimal invasive gynecological surgery, no one will agree-upon definition of "mini-laparotomy" but in general, a small abdominal incision can be used to extract uterine tissue [37 AAGL] (Level III). This can be performed using an LESS incision by extending a trocar incision or by making an incision in another location (e.g. Pfannenstiel or suprapubic).

A circumferential self-retaining retractor can be used to provide an expanded area for retrieval through these small incisions. The size and location of these types of incisions may have different risks such as infection and incisional hernia.

Reports of minilaparotomy incisions as small as 4 cm have demonstrated feasibility for the safe management of adnexal masses, myomectomy, benign hysterectomy and endometrial cancer.[6]

This also allows for hand-assisted dissection and suturing while retaining many benefits of a minimally invasive procedure.[7]

It should be noted that both vaginal and abdominal extirpation of a myoma have been associated with tissue dissemination if uncontained morcellation is performed. Accordingly, using a tissue retrieval bag to isolate specimens during this type of morcellation has been suggested.[8] The tissue is placed in a bag and brought to the anterior abdominal wall or vaginal orifice for manual morcellation with a scalpel or scissors within the bag.

In experienced hands, this method appears to be an efficient method to remove even large specimens.[8]

Intracorporeal Electromechanical Morcellation

Electromechanical morcellation (EMM, also known as "electronic" morcellation, "electric-generated" morcellation, and "power" morcellation) is a specific subtype of morcellation in which tissue is mobilized through a spinning or electrosurgical blade to cut it into smaller strips (AAGL). The tissue morcellator was first used by Kurt Semm in 1973.[9] Further, electromechanical power morcellators were approved by the US Food and Drug Administration (FDA) in 1995.

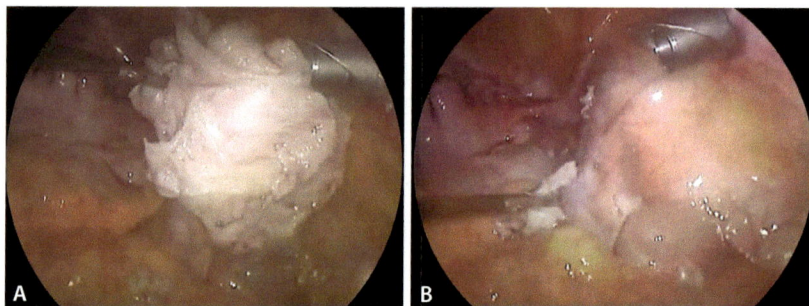

Figs. 1A and B: (A) Intraperitoneal power morcellation; (B) Fragments of tissue lying in the peritoneal cavity scattered after morcellation.

A variety of morcellators approved by the FDA for use in uterine surgery are available, featuring differences in blade diameter, cutting speed, weight, morcellation rate and mechanism of action. All existing morcellator devices employ either a laparoscopic port or are passed through a 12–20 mm laparoscopic incision.

Although their small blade diameter can result in a prolonged morcellation time to extract large tissue specimens, data suggest that some morcellator devices may work more efficiently than others[10] (AAGL) (Level III). Specifically, those having motor-peeling features demonstrate the fastest potential morcellation capabilities[11] (AAGL) (Level I).

Device-specific comparisons related to patient safety, risk of spread of an undetected uterine malignancy and intraperitoneal tissue fragment dissemination in general is lacking. There are no data to suggest any one device is associated with higher risk than another and surgeon experience is probably the most significant factor related to morcellator-related injuries[12] (AAGL) (Level III).

RISKS ASSOCIATED WITH INTRACORPOREAL MORCELLATION

Electromechanical morcellators have come under scrutiny regarding iatrogenic dissemination of benign and malignant tissue with fragments being inadvertently scattered during intracorporeal morcellation of leiomyomas, endometriosis, adenomyosis, splenic and ovarian tissues as well as occult uterine malignancies such as adenocarcinomas and sarcomas.[13,14]

Iatrogenic dissemination of malignant cells by morcellation has been shown to worsen the prognosis of patients with unsuspected sarcomas, increasing odds of tumor recurrence and death. Additionally, patients may require surgical re-exploration or chemotherapy that may have been unnecessary if tissue had been removed en bloc.[15]

Morcellated surgical specimens can be more difficult for pathologists to interpret than an intact specimen. With disruption of architecture, a tumor's original size and invasion may not be accurately determined and staging may be incorrect; focal areas of malignancy may be missed altogether.[16]

Iatrogenic complications from dissemination of benign tissue fragments implanting on parts of the abdominal cavity have resulted in peritonitis, intra-abdominal abscesses and intestinal obstruction. Case reports have described iatrogenic myomas on the appendix, bladder and retroperitoneally[14]; scattered leiomyomatosis throughout the pelvis has been reported.[17] The inadvertent spread of unrecognized malignant tissue is particularly concerning.

In response, in April 2014, the US FDA released a statement discouraging the use of laparoscopic power morcellation during hysterectomy or myomectomy.[18] In November 2014, the US FDA stated that power morcellation is contraindicated in peri- or postmenopausal women or women who are candidates for en bloc-specimen removal. In addition, a black box warning on power morcellators was released.

In a recent meta-analysis, the estimated rate of leiomyosarcoma was 0.51 per 1000 procedures or approximately 1 in 2000; restricting the meta-analysis to the 64 prospective studies resulted in a substantially lower estimate of 0.12 leiomyosarcomas per 1000 procedures or approximately 1 leiomyosarcoma per 8,300 surgeries.[19]

Withdrawing morcellation and not giving the benefits of laparoscopic surgery especially in young infertile women with fibroids or laparoscopic hysterectomy in patients with low risk of sarcomas are debatable. If uterine sarcoma is present, it will spread during every step of surgery whether it is open or laparoscopic. Malignant cells may spread while injecting vasopressin, during dissection and enucleation of myoma or during handling of specimen in peritoneal cavity. In bag morcellation, per se will not change prognosis of patient significantly.

In response to the US FDA's statements and low incidence of sarcoma, several reports of power morcellation in a contained isolation system (i.e., an insufflated bag), have demonstrated feasibility.[20]

In Bag Morcellation

Intracorporeal electromechanical morcellator use within a laparoscopic bag has been offered as a method to reduce tissue seeding in peritoneal cavity.[21] With this technique, the specimen is placed in a bag intraperitoneally and morcellation occurs with an electromechanical device in the confines of the bag. This promising method should mitigate iatrogenic tissue dissemination.

▪ TECHNIQUE

The steps of laparoscopic myomectomy and laparoscopic hysterectomy remain the same as done in a standardized fashion leaving the fibroid or uterus separated in the peritoneal cavity. The lower port on surgeon's side is

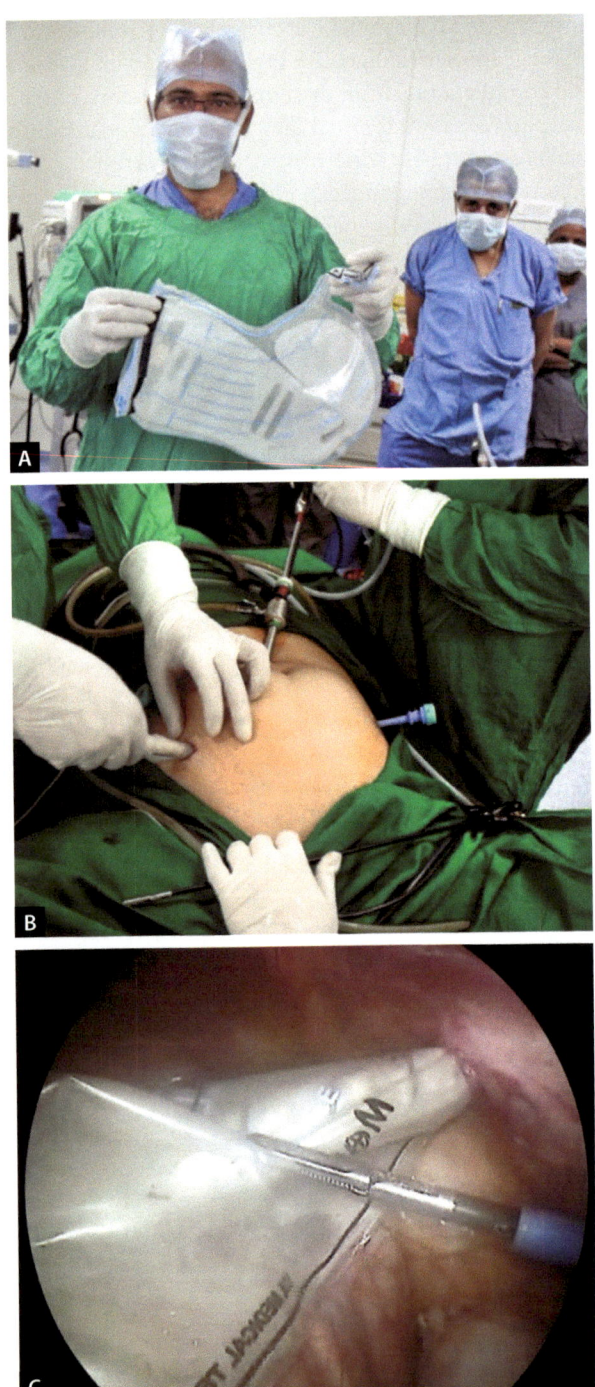

Figs. 2A to C

Myoma Specimen Retrieval Methods

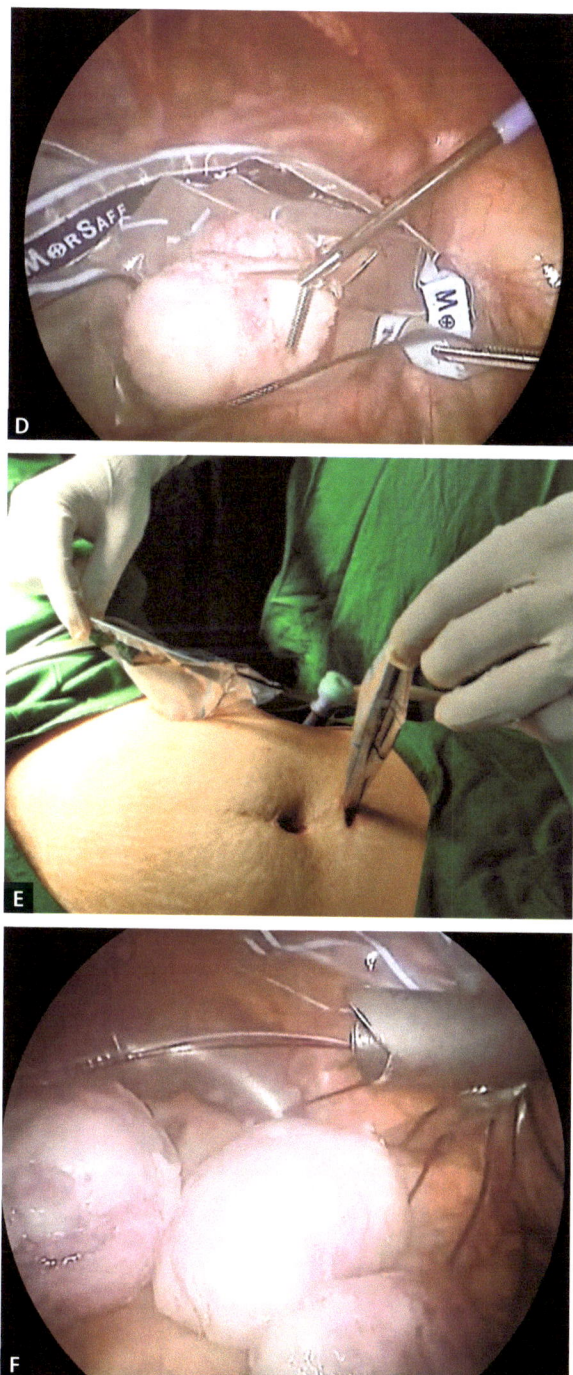

Figs. 2D to F

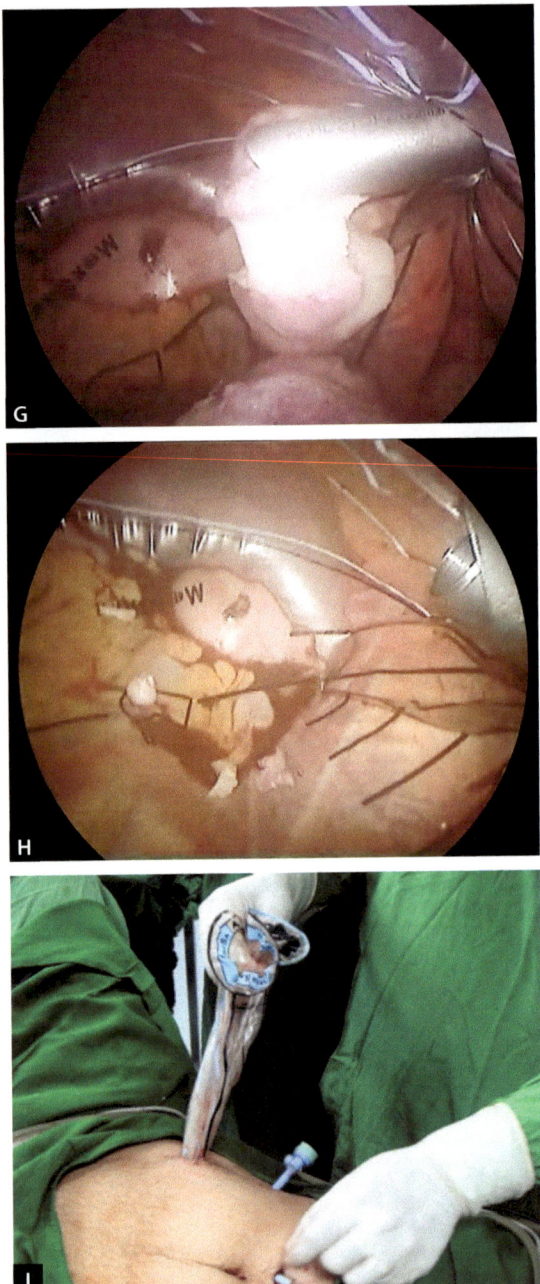

Figs. 2G to I
Figs. 2A to I: (A) Morcellation bag; (B to E) Steps of insertion of bag; (F) Fragments of myopia tissue within the morcellation bag; (G) In-bag morcellation; (H and I) Removal of bag

widened and mechanically stretched to make easy passage of the soft plastic sleeve carrying the bag. Depending on the size of the myoma specimen the bag size is selected. Different types of bags are available from different companies with little modifications.

Basically the bags have the shape like stomach with one wide opening called mouth for placement of specimen and later on morcellator blade. Other long narrow part of the bag is called tail which is used for placement of primary port and insufflation.

Placement of Bag

The wide opening of the bag is folded in a plastic sleeve and introduced inside the peritoneal cavity through the widened lower port under laparoscopic vision. Once the bag is placed in the peritoneal cavity the sleeve is removed, bag is unfolded and maneuvered such that mouth lies towards the lower morcellator port and tail directs towards primary port. 10 mm port with 5 mm reducer is placed through the lower port. The myoma is placed inside the bag and two parts of the opening of the bag are held together and pulled out withdrawing the 10-mm trocar. And then holding the two margins of the mouth, the bag is mechanically pulled by two hands of the surgeon bringing the entire mouth of the bag outside the lower port. Now from the lower port of opposite side, with a 5-mm grasper, the tail of the bag is held at the tip and railroaded inside the 10-mm primary port. The primary port is withdrawn and tail of the bag is brought outside the peritoneal cavity. The opening of the tail is widened to accommodate 10 mm primary port. The 10 mm primary port is placed inside the opening on the tail of bag and reintroduced inside the peritoneal cavity, laparoscope introduced and insufflation started. Now the myoma specimen lies inside the bag and bag completely lines the peritoneal cavity.

Once everything is in place, a 12-mm morcellator hand piece with a blunt tip trocar is introduced under vision inside the bag through the mouth of the bag. A 10-mm single tooth grasper is introduced inside the morcellator, which will hold the specimen and morcellation is done under vision as usual. With a series of long strips, the whole specimen is morcellated.

The bag at the end of morcellation contains the small bits of morcellated remnant pieces and the blood of specimen. The morcellator hand piece is removed blocking the mouth of the bag to prevent unnecessary scatter of tissue or fluid. The 10-mm trocar along with laparoscope are removed.

A knot is tied on the tail of the bag. The bag is pulled out from the morcellator port site, the tail end goes inside abdominal cavity and the complete bag is removed out from the morcellator port. The 10-mm port with laparoscope is reintroduced from the umbilical port and complete examination of the peritoneal cavity is done to confirm hemostasis. Port closure is done with suitable method.

Technical Difficulties

Sometimes placement of the bag can be cumbersome and difficult in initial cases. This can be overcome by mimicking the steps outside the peritoneal cavity. Twisting of the bag inside the peritoneal cavity should be avoided. Morcellator insertion should be gentle to avoid puncture of the bag.

INFORMED CONSENT: A RISK-SHARING PROCESS

Informed consent is a process of information sharing between surgeon and patient regarding risks, benefits and alternatives regarding a specific procedure. With all forms of tissue morcellation, the risks of dissemination of malignant and benign tissue in the peritoneal cavity and related health consequences and re-operation or additional treatments if needed should be explained to the patient. Also patient should be explained of missing of malignancy by pathologist due to disruption of tissue architecture.

These risks and the benefits of a minimally invasive approach as well as the risks and benefits of expectant management or laparotomy as alternatives should be explained. The risks of laparotomy should be noted.

A CRITICAL APPRAISAL OF THE SARCOMA AND MORCELLATION LITERATURE (AAGL)

- All studies regarding uterine leiomyosarcoma (LMS) outcomes in the setting of morcellation are single-institution and retrospective, and more than half of them contain fewer than 1000 patients.
- Most studies were conducted at high-volume academic medical or cancer centers. The incidence of uterine pathology and rare tumor types such as LMS tend to be higher in academic medical centers and may not reflect cancer incidence rates in the general population.
- Additionally, many of these studies were not stratified by sarcoma risk factors. Whether all candidates underwent a comprehensive preoperative evaluation and were appropriate candidates for a minimally invasive procedure remain unclear.
- However, several of the reports suggested that many of the women who underwent morcellation were menopausal and that rate of uterine LMS increased sharply with increasing age. Therefore, one should be particularly careful when considering morcellation in postmenopausal women, especially if the presumed preoperative diagnosis is uterine fibroids.

Prospective and population-based studies are needed to develop a better understanding of morcellator safety in different patient cohorts (e.g., women with large fibroids planning laparoscopic hysterectomy or myomectomy versus women with pelvic organ prolapse planning laparoscopic supracervical hysterectomy and sacrocolpopexy) and identify a population of women undergoing uterine surgery who may be at high risk of an unrecognized uterine cancer.

FUTURE DIRECTIONS

- For safe removal of specimens and to avoid harm to the patient, proper clinical collaboration with device manufacturing companies
- To develop better diagnostic methods for diagnosing uterine sarcoma preoperatively
- To report adverse events and device surveillance by professional societies, device manufacturing companies and regulatory system like FDA
- To maintain nationwide prospective surgical database of uterine surgeries
- A system for timely dissemination of hazards and concerns regarding devices and procedural complications
- Timely educational update and hands-on training regarding safe tissue extraction

The implementation of new technologies in minimal invasive gynecology should be patient centered with respect to safety and quality of life.

RECOMMENDATIONS (AAGL 2014) GUIDELINES ABOUT MORCELLATION

- Morcellation should not be used in the setting of known malignant or premalignant conditions.
- Morcellation should only be considered in patients if the appropriate evaluation of the myometrium, cervix and endometrium (with or without fibroids) is reassuring.
- For patients in whom malignancy is suspected preoperatively, alternatives to morcellation should be employed, including laparotomy.
- As the risk of malignancy, including undetectable malignancy, is increased in postmenopausal women, alternatives to morcellation should be considered in this patient population.
- When electromechanical morcellation (EMM) is planned, an informed consent should be taken. Patient autonomy must be respected.
- The use of morcellation within bag requires significant skill and experience and the use of specimen retrieval pouches should be investigated further for safety and outcomes in a controlled setting.

CONCLUSION

As the incidence of uterine sarcoma is very rare, benefits of electromechanical morcellation to young patients should be provided. Every attempt should be made to preoperatively suspect and diagnose the uterine sarcoma, though it is not always possible.

American Association of Gynecologic Laparoscopists (AAGL) stated that all existing methods of tissue extraction have benefits and risks, which must be balanced with maximizing benefits while minimizing harm to patients. As there is no single method that can protect all patients; therefore, all current methods of tissue extraction should remain available.

Gynecologic surgeons should actively discuss the risks of intracorporeal morcellation with their patients.

REFERENCES

AAGL Advancing Minimally Invasive Gynecology Worldwide, Morcellation During Uterine Tissue Extraction. The Tissue Extraction Task Force report, May 2014.

1. Nieboer TE, Johnson N, Lethaby A, et al. Surgical approach to hysterectomy for benign gynaecological disease. Cochrane Database System Rev. 2009;3.
2. Ghezzi F, Cromi A, Uccella S, Bogani G, Serati M, Bolis P. Transumbilical versus transvaginal retrieval of surgical specimens at laparoscopy: a randomized trial. Am J Obstet Gynecol. 2012;207:112.e1–112.e6.
3. Kho KA, Shin JH, Nezhat C. Vaginal extraction of large uteri with the Alexis retractor. J Minim Invasive Gynecol. 2009; 16:616-7.
4. Uccella S, Cromi A, Bogani G, Casarin J, Serati M, Ghezzi F. Transvaginal specimen extraction at laparoscopy without concomitant hysterectomy: our experience and systematic review of the literature. J Minim Invasive Gynecol. 2013;20:583-90
5. Kumar A, Pearl M. Mini-laparotomy versus laparoscopy for gynecologic conditions. J Minim Invasive Gynecol. 2014;21(1):109-14.
6. Alessandri F, Lijoi D, Mistrangelo E, Ferrero S, Ragni N. Randomized study of laparoscopic versus minilaparotomic myomectomy for uterine myomas. J Minim Invasive Gynecol; 2006
7. Serur E, Lakhi N. Tips and tricks for successful manual morcellation: a response to "vaginal morcellation: a new strategy for large gynecological malignant tumor extraction". Gynecol Oncol. 2013;128:150.
8. Favero G, Anton C, Silva e Silva A, Ribeiro A, Araujo MP, Miglino G, et al. Vaginal morcellation: a new strategy for large gynecological malignant tumor extraction: a pilot study. Gynecol Oncol. 2012;126:443-7.
9. Semm K. Morcellement and suturing using pelviscopy: not a problem anymore [in German]. Geburtshilfe Frauenheilkd.1991;51:843-6.
10. Carter JE, McCarus SD. Laparoscopic myomectomy. Time and cost analysis of power vs. manual morcellation. J Reprod Med 1997 Jul;42(7):383-388.
11. Zullo F, Falbo A, Iuliano A, Oppedisano R, Sacchinelli A, Annunziata G, et al. Randomized controlled study comparing the Gynecare Morcellex and Rotocut G1 tissue morcellators. J Minim Invasive Gynecol. 2010;17(2):192-9.
12. Milad MP, Milad EA. Laparoscopic morcellator-related complications. J Minim Invasive Gynecol; 2013.
13. Kho KA, Nezhat C. Parasitic myomas. Obstet Gynecol. 2009;114:611-5.
14. Al-Talib A, Tulandi T. Pathophysiology and possible iatrogenic cause of leiomyomatosis peritonealis disseminata. Gynecol Obstet Invest. 2010;69:239-44.

15. Oduyebo T, Rauh-Hain AJ, Meserve EE, Seidman MA, Hinchcliff E, George S, et al. The value of re-exploration in patients with inadvertently morcellated uterine sarcoma. Gynecol Oncol. 2014;132:360-5.
16. Rivard C, Salhadar A, Kenton K. New challenges in detecting, grading, and staging endometrial cancer after uterine morcellation. J Minim Invasive Gynecol. 2012;19:313-6.
17. Takeda A, Mori M, Sakai K, Mitsui T, Nakamura H. Parasitic peritoneal leiomyomatosis diagnosed 6 years after laparoscopic myomectomy with electric tissue morcellation: report of a case and review of the literature. J Minim Invasive Gynecol. 2007;14:770-5.
18. US Food and Drug Administration. Laparoscopic Uterine Power Morcellation in Hysterectomy and Myomectomy. FDA Safety Communication. Silver Spring, MD: USFDA; 2014.
19. Pritts EA, Vanness DJ. The prevalence of occult leiomyosarcoma at surgery for presumed uterine fibroids: a meta-analysis. Gynecol Surg. 2015;12:165-77.
20. Einarsson JI, Cohen SL, Fuchs N, Wang KC. In-bag morcellation. J Minim Invasive Gynecol. 2014;21:951-3.
21. Sinha RY, Joshi KM, Warty NR, Frey B. Morcellation in the bag: the superior solution to avoid spillage. Gynaecol Endosc. 2000;9:103-6.